Secrets to my Hypothyroidism Success:

A Personal Guide to Hypothyroidism Freedom

Welcome Letter:

As humans we are troubled by so many things. Sometimes, when I sit down to write, I have no idea what I am going to say. I start to begin anyways on a blank word document and eventually the words start following right out of my fingertips where it's hard for me to keep up. As I am writing, I think about the women who will read my written work and become inspired, what has brought them to this point in their life and I often wonder how this will bless her and help her in her life. Honestly, everything that I write, I start out writing it for myself.

My new purpose is to empower people to embrace who they are, to add value to their life, to inspire them and to connect with those who are struggling with hypothyroidism. You need to realize that you have to invest in your health. You are worth investing money into yourself and take charge of your health. Will it "hurt" a little? Ha, you bet, but it will change your life.

I wish somebody had given me a step-by-step road-map back when I was first diagnosed with hypothyroidism. The solutions in this book has helped so many people. I've done my best to pull from all their expertise, as well as my own knowledge and clinical experience. I want to make it easy for you to find the answers quickly, all in the one place, because I'm all too familiar with that awful side effects of hypothyroidism. I certainly don't want you to have to spend years finding solutions, like I did. I also want you to understand that there isn't an easy "one pill" solution, but the "one pill" approach that our current medical system is using is NOT WORKING because the underlying cause for hypothyroidism is not being addressed.

Knowledge is power, educate yourself and find the answer to your health care needs. Wisdom is a wonderful thing to seek. I hope this book will teach and encourage you to take leaps in your life to educate yourself for a happier & healthier life. You have to take ownership of your health

The best patient to be is a well informed and an educated patient. My blogs and books can make the difference between you having the energy to live your life as you want, or merely dragging yourself through life.

Just think how great it's going to feel when you are as healthy on the inside as you look on the outside! The ultimate goal isn't to look fit but to be fit.

Your most powerful tool to change your health is your fork.

May abundant Health, Wealth and Blessings be yours,

A.L. Childers

xoxo

This book thanks everyone suffering from hypothyroidism and looking for answers and for all the nutritionists, holistic health professionals and medical professionals who are making a difference in the field of nutrition and hypothyroidism.

A lack of knowledge is a lack of power.

Disclaimer

The information and recipes contained in this book are based upon the research and the personal experiences of the author. It's for entertainment purposes only. It is not meant to replace any advice from a health care professional. This book is meant to compliment. The reader is encouraged to use good judgement when apply the information contained and to seek advice from a qualified professional if, and as, needed. Every attempt has been made to provide accurate, up to date and reliable information. No warranties of any kind are expressed or implied. Readers acknowledge that the author is not engaging in the rendering of legal, financial, medical or professional advice. By reading this, the reader agrees that under no circumstance the author is not responsible for any loss, direct or indirect, which are incurred by using this information contained within this book. Including but not limited to errors, omissions or inaccuracies. This book is not intended as replacements from what your health care provider has suggested. The author is not responsible for any adverse effects or consequences resulting from the use of any of the suggestions, preparations or procedures discussed in this book. All matters pertaining to your health should be supervised by a health care professional. I am not a doctor, or a medical professional. This book is designed for as an educational and entertainment tool only. Please always check with your health practitioner before taking any vitamins, supplements, diet change, or herbs, as they may have side-effects, especially when combined with medications, alcohol, or other vitamins or supplements. Knowledge is power, educate yourself and find the answer to your health care needs. Wisdom is a wonderful thing to seek. I hope this book will teach and encourage you to take leaps in your life to educate yourself for a happier & healthier life. You have to take ownership of your health. All rights reserved. No part of this publication may be reproduced, distributed, or transmitted in any form or by any means, including photo copying, or recording, or other electronic, or mechanical methods, without the prior written permission of the author, except in the case of brief quotations, embodied in critical reviews, in certain other noncommercial uses permitted by copyright laws. Although every precaution has been taken by the author to verify the accuracy of the information contained herein, the author assumes no responsibility for any errors, or omissions. No liability is assumed for damages that may result from the information that is obtained within.

A.L. Childers

Thanks for reading my latest book. Please let me know if you need any support with it.

A note of caution:

I strongly support self-care, personal health empowerment and improving your understanding of thyroid health. However, this cannot substitute by a trained medical professional in cases of long standing and undiagnosed symptoms. This book is thus not meant as a substitute for professional medical judgement, though it can serve as a helpful adjunct to it. All content within this book is commentary or opinion and is protected under Free Speech laws in all the civilized world. The information herein is provided for educational and entertainment purposes only

When in doubt about your thyroid seek your doctor or your medical professional to exclude serious medical conditions. It is not intended as a substitute for professional advice of any kind. Audrey Childers assumes no responsibility for the use or misuse of this material.

Therefore no warranty of any kind, whether expressed or implied, is given in relation to this information. This is a comprehensive limitation of liability that applies to all damages of any kind, including (without limitation) compensatory; direct, indirect or consequential damages; loss of data, income or profit; loss of or damage to property and claims of third parties.

Be safe, be sane and be healthy.

Get a complete exam from a reliable health practitioner. Do what you can do within the boundaries of good common sense.

In a word, be kind to yourself and your thyroid.

Your Personal Contract

I...

Declare that I will master my life in every aspect of it. I will no longer settle for less than I deserve. I have the courage, will power and wisdom to know that it's my time to make a difference in my life. I will put my best foot forward in all areas of my life. I will wake up grateful, put the right foods in my body for nourishment and uplift others.

I am the only person responsible for my life and I believe with every fiber of my being that that I can make a difference.

I am enough. I will be true to myself and follow my heart. My personal development is in my own hands AND I will stop fighting against myself. I will stop listening to self-doubt. My past experiences will not affect my current mindset. God will support me in with joyful abundance in all areas of my life. This book is only the beginning of my wonderful journey to happiness, joy, peace and prosperity. I am willing to go beyond my past and I am the only person who chooses my path and I don't need anyone's approval. I release all limitations from my past.

I will seek the highest truth and the most healing ways to live my life.   Health and Happiness is abundantly mine.

Love,

Signed by ....

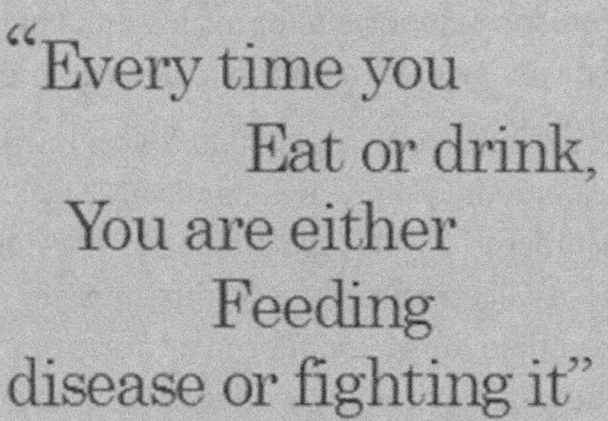

"Every time you
Eat or drink,
You are either
Feeding
disease or fighting it"

Introduction:

Around 20 million Americans and 250 million people worldwide will be affected by low thyroid function or hypothyroidism. One in 8 women will struggle with a thyroid problem in her lifetime, and up to 90% of all thyroid problems are autoimmune in nature, the most common of which is Hashimoto's. Many people don't know that hypothyroidism is an autoimmune disease and the reason why most doctors don't mention is because it's simple: it doesn't affect their treatment plan. Traditional medicine treats autoimmune disorders with steroids and other methods that suppress the immune system. The number of people suffering from hypothyroidism continues to rise each year. Levothyroxine is the 4th highest selling drug in the U.S. Every Cell in your body responds to your thyroid hormones. These hormones have a direct impact on every major system in your body.

Hypothyroidism is the kind of disease that carries a bit of mystery with it. This book is not for readers looking for quick answers. There is not one size fits all. You have to be in charge of your health. I didn't write this book to sell you any "snake oil" in a bottle. I've written this book to be an eye opener for you and to share with you what I have learned on my journey. The solutions in this book has helped so many people. There are many incredible holistic practitioners, authors and researchers with experience and expertise in this area. I've done my best to pull from all their expertise, as well as my own knowledge and clinical experience. I want to make it easy for you to find the answers quickly, all in the one place, because I'm all too familiar with that awful side effects of hypothyroidism. I certainly don't want you to have to spend years finding solutions, like I did. I also what you to understand that there isn't an easy "one pill" solution, but the "one pill" approach that our current medical system is using is NOT WORKING because the underlying cause for hypothyroidism is not being addressed. Many people never question their doctors, research their medications or find out the side effects of what was prescribed. Don't misconstrue what I am saying being on medication isn't a bad thing when it is necessary but sometimes the medications that are given will camouflage the real symptoms. The problem with giving people thyroid hormone is that it may not be addressing the root cause of your hypothyroidism. If you start addressing the root cause your body will start to heal itself. All these years of bad eating habits beginning in your childhood, a stressful life, lack of exercise/too much exercise, environmental toxins and little to no sleep have contributed to your hypothyroidism. So many of us have these crazy phantom-like health problems. The best patient to be is a well informed and an educated patient. This book can make the difference between you having the energy to live your life as you want, or merely dragging yourself through life. Don't be upset with your medical doctor or endocrinologist they are there to treat your illness not really to give advice on getting to the root of the cause. These doctors are needed. A Health Practitioner will get to the root of your cause and start helping you heal yourself from the main underlying issues. In this book, you will learn the link that ties many of our issues together. Get ready to go on a journey of discovery where you are going to learn how everything ties into one. The foods we eat can interfere with your thyroid medication. Our body is lacking certain nutrients that heavily influence the function of our thyroid gland while certain foods can inhibit your body's ability to absorb the replacement hormones. There is no one size fits all program when you are dealing with hypothyroidism. When you start to eat smarter and are aware of what foods feed your body, despite the condition, you can start to feel better and manage your symptoms. In this age of overly processed, genetically modified, artificially flavored and preservative loaded foods.

I'm very excited that you bought this book and are wanting to find an answer to what is hindering your life. Think about this. Americans are in such a pathetic health crisis. We have the abundance of everything at our finger tips but yet we 1 in 3 people are on some sort of medication. It doesn't matter if it's Prescribed or over the counter. Meanwhile billions of people around the world are in better health than the average American, doesn't have to be on some sort of medication and are in their correct body mass index. We are in such a state of denial. My mission is to do everything in my power to help you to start healing and reach your fullest potential. To help be a source of inspiration you seek and attract what you desire with the faith that your vision of success is your destiny! You deserve to kick yourself out of that fat storage unhealthy mode and into a fat burning healthy mode. Remember, what we eat, governs what we become.

Dedication:

I dedicate this book to one of my best friends, Tanja. Whom I've shared a million laughs with, you know all my stories and most of them you help me write. I hope we will always be friends and continue writing our friendship story.

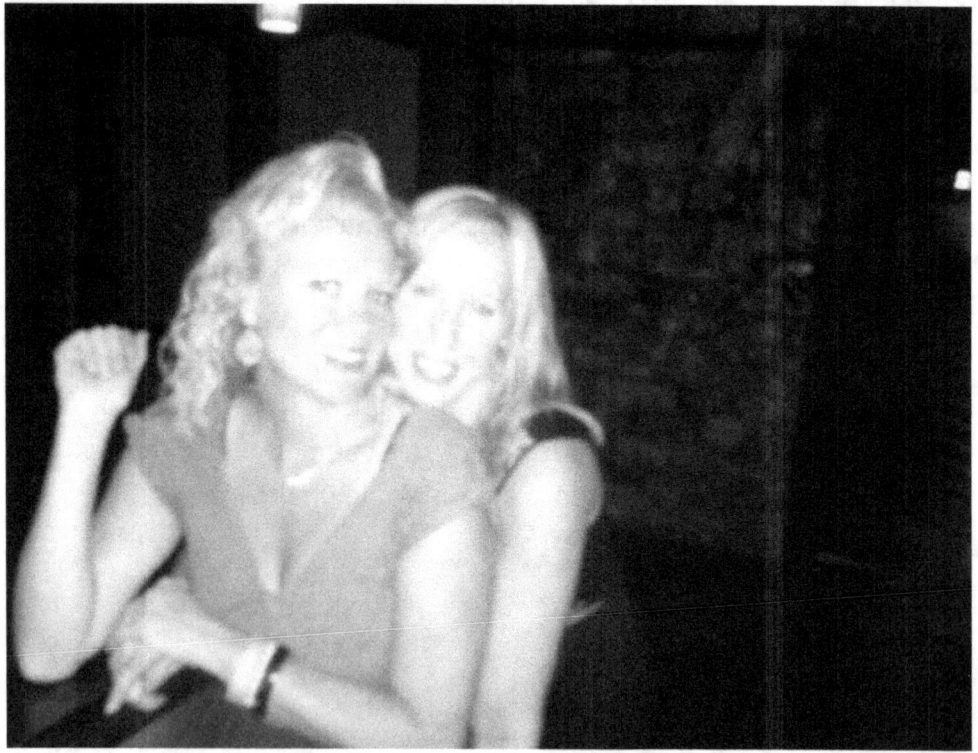

A note of caution:

I strongly support self-care, personal health empowerment and improving your understanding of thyroid health. However, this cannot substitute by a trained medical professional in cases of long standing and undiagnosed symptoms. This book is thus not meant as a substitute for professional medical judgement, though it can serve as a helpful adjunct to it.

When in doubt about your thyroid seek your doctor or your medical professional to exclude serious medical conditions.

Be safe, be sane and be healthy.

Get a complete exam from a reliable health practitioner. Do what you can do within the boundaries of good common sense.

In a word, be kind to yourself and your thyroid.

Author Note:

Let's not forget that we are all different. Each one of us are unique and we are biochemically individually wired and what works for one person may not work for another. We are extremely complex and each person should be valued independently. My reason for having hypothyroidism might not be your reason. Hypothyroidism isn't a 1 size fits all solution. I want to try to help you understand the many debilitating aspects of this medical condition. This book is packed full of repetitive information and is meant to be an eye opener for everyone who wants to make a difference in their lives and what some doctors just won't tell you. I want this book to be just one of your resources that is empowering to try to help you make sense of it all. We need our medical doctors, health practitioners and those who have studied years but I urge you to also find another doctor if your doctor won't listen to you or even allow you to see your lab results or even if you doctor refuses to perform necessary needed lab work.

My story

After being diagnosed with hypothyroidism over 25 years ago. I knew there was something more than just being labeled with a medical condition. There wasn't a lot of information on how to heal myself.

I felt as if I had lost control over my body and my mental health as well. It seems that I had experienced every symptom from lack of energy, anxiety, weight gain, scary heart palpitations and brain fog. I couldn't sleep and where the hell had my eye brows gone? My hair loss was thinning, I was always constipated, my blood pressure started to increase, my fingertips would get cold and numb just out of the blue, my emotions were all over the place, I was on an emotional roller coaster. I had aches and pains that it seemed hard to explain to my doctor and my doctor thought it was all in my head. My doctor wanted to give me thyroid medication plus antidepressants. I was not depressed. The simplest tasks seemed like the hardest on some days. I really didn't realize or understand the whole life impact that my "new" condition, because as I started investigating I realized that all the wide ranging symptoms of hypothyroidism were being brushed off by my doctor at the time as being part of everyday life, stress or getting older.

After being diagnosis, I was relieved and excited to finally have an answer, some kind of answer, to what was going on with my body but soon I was disappointed again only to find out that the thyroid medications that I thought was going bring you back to myself only fixed a few of my symptoms and I was still having to deal with a dozen more remaining issues. I was so tired of hearing that it was all in my head. I wanted to scream to the world and let everyone know that my quality of life had drastically been affected and there has to be answers.

Somewhere, Someone, Anyone at this point, hello? Help me, I feel like I am drowning, slowly dying and the world just keeps turning. Why isn't anyone listening to me?

My quality of life has been affected.

Every Cell in my body responds to the foods that I eat, the products that I put on my body to the house hold chemicals that I purchase for my home. All of these things have a direct impact on my hormones and in return my hormones have a direct impact on every major system in my body. Not to mention that my body was lacking certain nutrients that heavily influence the function of every cell in my body.

The foods that I consume, oh, the foods I consume.

I've learned in my journey that organic, whole, nutrient rich food is medicine. I really can't say it any simpler than that. There is a major disconnect between what we believe to be healthy foods and what research tells us is healthy. In fact, many of the health foods today that people go out of their way to eat daily are extremely thyroid suppressive.

I started to become my very own health investigator. I started researching what I need to do to start addressing what the root cause that lead to me to this point in my life. I certainly wouldn't take Motrin if I got a pebble stuck in my shoe? So, why am I going to take this new medication for my thyroid if I didn't understand how I got here?

As I began researching I soon discovered that hypothyroidism does has a root issue. I often ignored all the underlying causes of my hypothyroidism. What was I looking for? Like an onion, I needed to see it layer by layer. I started to do a little pruning of my branches, I wanted to be healthy again. My thyroid was being influenced by many so many different things.

You see, the main problem with hypothyroidism is that it's a very tricky condition and complicated disorder to manage. There is no one size fits all program when you are dealing with hypothyroidism.

Around 20 million Americans and 250 million people worldwide will be affected by low thyroid function or hypothyroidism. One in 8 women will struggle with a thyroid problem in her lifetime, and up to 90% of all thyroid problems are autoimmune in nature, the most common of which is Hashimoto's. As diseases go, you would think that it would be a cinch to diagnose and pretty straightforward to treat. Many people don't know that hypothyroidism is an autoimmune disease and the reason why most doctors don't mention is because it's simple: it doesn't affect their treatment plan. Traditional medicine treats autoimmune disorders with steroids and other methods that suppress the immune system. The number of people suffering from hypothyroidism continues to rise each year. **Levothyroxine is the 4th highest selling drug in the U.S. THE 4TH HIGHEST SELLING DRUG!**

Every Cell in your body responds to your thyroid hormones. These hormones have a direct impact on every major system in your body.

As consumers we put our trust in the research and development of scientific studies, The FDA and The CDC. Drug store chains have quota's to meet and even some of our Doctors get yearly bonus's. Little do we do that behind closed doors corporations often pay scientists and these companies to support their product for profit. Some Politicians seem to have a revolving door between the private and public sector. The synthetic chemicals we face every day that is in our food, our water, and the air that we breathe.

Did you know that products we use every day may contain toxic chemicals and has been linked to women's health issues? They are hidden endocrine disruptors and are very tricky chemicals that play havoc on our bodies. "We are all routinely exposed to endocrine disruptors, and this has the potential to significantly harm the health of our youth," said Renee Sharp, EWG's director of research. "It's important to do what we can to avoid them, but at the same time we can't shop our way out of the problem. We need to have a real chemical policy reform. " The longer the length of ingredients on your food or body product labels means how much more unhealthy it is for you to consume or place on your body. When an item contains a host of ingredients that most likely you can't even pronounce or remember to spell you can bet your lucky dollar that the natural nutrients are long gone. These highly processed frank n foods or body products are very difficult for the body to break down and some of the chemicals will become stored in your body. Your body doesn't know how to process it, so it gets stored.

No wonder our bodies are completely bombarded and overwhelmed with the constant exposed to toxic chemicals through the air that we breathe, the water we drink, the foods we eat, and the personal care products and cleaning products we use.

After being diagnosed with hypothyroidism over 25 years ago. I knew there was something more than just being labeled with this medical condition. There certainly wasn't a whole lot of information on how to heal myself. Continuing my research I began to understand that there really isn't a one size fits all diet for everyone who is has been diagnosed with Hypothyroidism but there are certain ways you can eat that will certainly help begin the healing process. Diet alone isn't enough to help your body start fighting this battle that is raging in your body. The food you eat is your first line of defense against hypothyroidism. You must start addressing other areas in your life.

This was a lifestyle change that I needed to pursue not another fade diet.

My new purpose is to empower people to embrace who they are, to add value to their life, to inspire them and to connect with those who are struggling with hypothyroidism. You need to realize that you have to invest in your health. You are worth investing money into yourself and take charge of your health. Will it "hurt" a little? Ha, you bet, but it will change your life.

I wish somebody had given me a step-by-step road-map back when I was first diagnosed with hypothyroidism. The solutions in this book has helped so many people. I've done my best to pull from all their expertise, as well as my own knowledge and clinical experience. I want to make it easy for you to find the answers quickly, all in the one place, because I'm all too familiar with that awful side effects of hypothyroidism. I certainly don't want you to have to spend years finding solutions, like I did. I also want you to understand that there isn't an easy "one pill" solution, but the "one pill" approach that our current medical system is using is NOT WORKING because the underlying cause for hypothyroidism is not being addressed.

It's been many years since I started on this journey of discovery. I've written many articles, a ton of blogging on my website Thehypothyroidismchick.com and published 6 books. My goal is to educate those who are on a similar path as mine with hypothyroidism. Lately, there's been something very deep nudging at my very core screaming to come out. I finally decided to let it seep out of my fingertips into this book. When I began writing about hypothyroidism, I knew it was an uncharted territory. My mindset was to search the truth, share my experiences and write compelling articles. The more I write, the more polished I become to develop my palate and skill-set. I have found something that I deeply care about and its worth every-bit of cherishing.

I write from the heart and share my truth.

I've realized that there will always be people who will always be a follower and never a leader when it comes to their health or their life in general. You must analyze your own truths and never from someone else's perceptive , always be your own life advocate and form your own truths with your own ideas of what is going to work in your life.

What I express in my blogs, books and articles are purely my views and opinions from the research and readings that I've done. I do not claim to have the absolute entire truth; this is simply what I have concluded at this moment in my life.

As each passing day goes, I continue to learn. As each passing day goes, I continue to grow.

We all have our very own skills and talents that we have to offer the world. I encourage you to find yours.

Let's get on thing straight.

I'm not trying to sell your health. I am trying to open your eyes and give you a purpose to start being healthy.

There is no such thing as something for nothing. So many people don't listen to their bodies. If you are constantly putting the wrong gas in your car is will start to eventually break down. Your body is the same way. One of the most common failure is the habit of quitting. Don't allow this type of failure of defeat to trick you into quitting. You are worth great health. You have the abundance of good health within your reach.

Being healthy is a state of mind. When you start to realize that the food you eat, the products you use and the way you live all talk to your DNA. Once you realize that you have a choice to change and you want to change you will change. You will start to read labels, you will think about what you're eating, how it was made and will it benefit your body.

Impossible? No! Not at all.

Being healthy does come from those with a healthy conscious. You and you alone must decide whether or not good health is important. Is good health worth the effort? You see we are wiping ourselves out. It seems with all the bad choices we are ultimately preparing ourselves for our own final destruction's. We often do choose badly but it's our choice to do so. The diet industry is a load of bullshit. Eat less, exercise more doesn't work. None of us should be on the same eating plan. What I mean by this is, each of us are unique. I may be allergic to eggs or dairy or gluten whereas someone else isn't. I may be need to take more vitamin b or vitamin d where your body is adequately great. I may need to eat more potassium rich foods where your body could have a potassium abundance. Working with a Knowledgeable Health Practitioner will do the proper blood work and screenings to see what exactly your body needs.

The main reason why you should work with a knowledgeable health practitioner is its patient-centered medical healing at its best. Unfortunately when it comes to hypothyroidism there isn't a one size fits all approach to dealing with it and often times you are left still searching for the answers to your symptoms when all you want is your zest for life back. A knowledgeable health practitioner will care for you as an individual as they won't look at your body as a whole they will treat each individual body symptom, imbalance and dysfunction. They certainly move from the confusion of the "one size fits all treatment" approach that we know isn't working to the one that will cater to what your body needs. Let's not forget that each of us are a unique case and unless you get a proper thorough clinical evaluation, trying to figure what medical advise you need online is dubious at best.

Imagine your body is one piece of machinery. Your entire body works together and if one area is affected it's like a domino effect on the other areas. It puts a strain on the other areas and they have to work harder to pull the weight of that area that not working like it should. So, start working on reducing your body's total load. Your health condition has a root cause. Once you start addressing the root of your problems is when your body can start healing itself. Your body is an awesome design but there is a complex balance between everything. It's a domino effect. Four things you must start doing immediately is getting your immune system in check, fixing your unhealthy gut, change your mindset and decrease your inflammation.   Inflammation disrupts the production and regulatory mechanisms of hormones. Remember what I've already said: Sometimes we have to do a little pruning of the branches, in order for the tree to be healthy again.

Why? We are all different.

Break that cycle today, start eating to cater to your thyroid and replenish your life. Knowledge is power, educate yourself and find the answer to your health care needs. Wisdom is a wonderful thing to seek. I hope this book will teach and encourage you to take leaps in your life to educate yourself for a happier & healthier life.

You have the power to make a difference in your life. You've always had the power. No one can force you to become more aware of what you put on your body and what you put in your body. What you eat is just as important as what you put on your body. Adjusting your life, reading labels and catering to your specific health needs isn't easy but it will benefit you in the long run. This is one of the smartest decisions that you can make. Not only will you start to look and feel better but think of the medical cost that you could be saving your future self.

The Real Story behind Hypothyroidism

Fact: Every Cell in your body responds to your thyroid hormones. These hormones have a direct impact on every major system in your body.

Hypothyroidism is a consequence of actions taken. It is a combination of sequences that you allowed to take place to get you to this point in your life. Yes, I am pointing the finger at you. I am pointing the finger at myself. I am so busy of "not being aware" and" grabbing what is easy" that I've allowed this to happen. There is this big lie that we all got stuck in.   Listen to me when I say there's a major disconnect between what YOU believe to be healthy foods and what research tells us is healthy. In fact, many of the health foods today that people go out of their way to eat daily are extremely thyroid suppressive.

As diseases go, you would think that it would be a cinch to diagnose and pretty straightforward to treat. Each of us are unique individuals with different sensitivities. None of has the same exact routine as far as what foods we eat, what chemicals we are exposed to and what medications we take but yet we all are similar when it comes to our thyroids not working properly.

First, please give me a moment to explain how the thyroid works.

Hypothyroidism means your thyroid is not making enough thyroid hormone. Your thyroid is a butterfly-shaped gland in the front of your throat. It makes the hormones that control the way your body uses energy. Basically, our thyroid hormone tells all the cells in our bodies how busy they should be.

Most doctors will prescribe you a synthetic version of thyroid hormone called Synthroid (levothyroxine). First introduced in 1959, Synthroid is the third most frequently prescribed drugs in the United States. For the sixty years prior to

Synthroid, the standard treatment was a desiccated (dried) concentrate of pig thyroid, which remains popular today, although not nearly as popular as its successor per Robert Rountree, M.D., who is a physician in private practice and an Herb Research Foundation advisory board member.

How were you diagnosed? Did your doctor just perform a simple TSH test and it showed that you had an elevated presence of thyroid stimulating hormone in your blood?

TSH is made in the pituitary, a small gland near the center of the brain. When the thyroid gland doesn't make enough T4, the pituitary increases its production of TSH in an attempt to make the gland work harder. In other words, thyroid hormone production is regulated by a simple negative feedback loop. When a diseased gland fails to make enough T4, the quick and easy solution is to replace it with a synthetic version. Per Robert Rountree, M.D., who is a physician in private practice and an Herb Research Foundation advisory board member.

Hold on. Don't be so quick to start taking that synthetic version of T4 only medication. Synthetics like thyroxine will eventually destroy the thyroid where you will have to be on some form of thyroid medication for the rest of your life. Also, everything that glitters isn't gold. There isn't a one size fits all solution to hypothyroidism. This is why you have to work with your doctor. Requests a full thyroid panel which should at least include these 6 key thyroid labs that are listed below. Some of us, need T3 along with our T4 medication because our T4 isn't converting into a must needed hormone called T3. This is why most people have partial improvements. Also, the conversion to T3 is affected by nutritional deficiencies such as low selenium, inadequate omega-3 fatty acids, low zinc, chemicals from the environment, or by stress. Further in the book, I will cover nutritional deficiencies, vitamins, exercise and other environmental factors.

Is your head spinning yet with all this information!

A full thyroid panel for hypothyroidism should at least include these key thyroid lab tests:

TSH

Free T4

Free T3

Reverse T3

Thyroid Peroxidase Antibodies

Thyroglobulin Antibodies

Listen TSH alone does not give a full picture of thyroid health.

Normal Ranges for you blood work

TSH- (range .034 – 4.82)

Free- T4 (range 0.59 – 1.17)

Total -T4 (range 4.5 – 12.0)

Total- T3 (range 71 – 180)

1. TSH (Thyroid Stimulating Hormone) TSH – This is a pituitary hormone that responds to low/high amounts of circulating thyroid hormone. In advanced cases of Hashimoto's and primary hypothyroidism, this lab test will be elevated, (read post about interpreting your TSH test). In the case of Graves' disease the TSH will be low. People with Hashimoto's and central hypothyroidism may have a normal reading on this test.

2. Thyroid peroxidase antibodies (TPO Antibodies) Thyroid peroxidase antibodies (TPO Antibodies) and Thyroglobulin Antibodies (TG Antibodies) – Most people with Hashimoto's will have an elevation of one or both of these antibodies. These

antibodies are often elevated for decades before a change in TSH is seen. People with Graves' disease and thyroid cancer may also have an elevation in thyroid antibodies including TPO & TG, as well as TSH receptor antibodies.

3. Thyroglobulin Antibodies (TG Antibodies) Read # 2

4. Thyroid Ultrasound Thyroid Ultrasound – A small percentage of people may have Hashimoto's, but may not have thyroid antibodies detectable in the blood. Doing a thyroid ultrasound will help your physician determine a diagnosis.

5. Free T3 Free T3 & Free T4 – These tests measure the levels of active thyroid hormone circulating in the body. When these levels are low, but your TSH tests in the normal range, this may lead your physician to suspect a rare type of hypothyroidism, known as central hypothyroidism.

6. Free T4

7. Reverse T3

You must be an advocate for health and insist on all the following tests especially the two thyroid antibody tests.

Thyroid Peroxidase Antibodies (TPOAb) #2

Thyroglobulin Antibodies (TgAb) #3

Don't allow your doctor to refuse to give you these tests. Many people have normal lab tests but still have Hashimoto's disease. It's all in the antibodies!

Environmental chemicals and toxins, pesticides, BPA, thyroid endocrine disruptors, iodine imbalance, other medications, fluoride, overuse of soy products, cigarette smoking, and gluten intolerance. All of these play a very important role in your thyroid health. A nonprofit group called Beyond Pesticides warns that some 60 percent of pesticides used today have been shown to affect the thyroid gland's production of T3 and T4 hormones. Commercially available insecticides and fungicides have also been involved. Even dental x-rays have been linked to an increased risk of thyroid disorders.

As consumers we put our trust in the research and development of scientific studies, The FDA and The CDC. Drug store chains have quota's to meet and even some of our Doctors get yearly bonus's. Little do we do that behind closed doors corporations often pay scientists and these companies to support their product for profit. Some Politicians seem to have a revolving door between the private and public sector. The synthetic chemicals we face every day that is in our food, our water, and the air that we breathe.

Did you know that products we use every day may contain toxic chemicals and has been linked to women's health issues? They are hidden endocrine disruptors and are very tricky chemicals that play havoc on our bodies. "We are all routinely exposed to endocrine disruptors, and this has the potential to significantly harm the health of our youth," said Renee Sharp, EWG's director of research. "It's important to do what we can to avoid them, but at the same time we can't shop our way out of the problem. We need to have a real chemical policy reform." The longer the length of ingredients on your food label means how much more unhealthy it is for you to consume. When an item contains a host of ingredients that most likely you can't even pronounce or remember to spell you can bet your lucky dollar that the natural nutrients are long gone. These highly processed frank n foods are very difficult for the body to break down and some of the chemicals will become stored in your body.

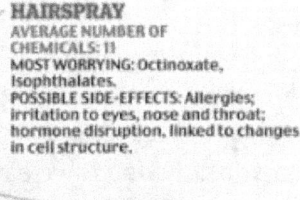

SHAMPOO
AVERAGE NUMBER OF CHEMICALS: 15
MOST WORRYING: Sodium Lauryl Sulphate; Tetrasodium and Propylene Glycol.
POSSIBLE SIDE-EFFECTS: Irritation; possible eye damage.

EYE SHADOW
CHEMICALS: 26
MOST WORRYING: Polythylene terephthalate.
POSSIBLE SIDE-EFFECTS: Linked to cancer; infertility; hormonal disruptions and damage to the body's organs.

LIPSTICK
CHEMICALS: 33
MOST WORRYING: Polymenthyl methacrylate.
POSSIBLE SIDE-EFFECTS: Allergies; links to cancer.

NAIL VARNISH
CHEMICALS: 31
MOST WORRYING: Phthalates.
POSSIBLE SIDE-EFFECTS: Linked to fertility issues and problems in developing babies.

PERFUME:
CHEMICALS: 250
MOST WORRYING: Benzaldehyde.
POSSIBLE SIDE-EFFECTS: Irritation to mouth, throat and eyes; nausea; linked to kidney damage.

FAKE TAN
CHEMICALS: 22
MOST WORRYING: Ethylparaben, Methylaparaben, Propylparaben.
POSSIBLE SIDE-EFFECTS: Rashes; irritation; hormonal disruption.

HAIRSPRAY
AVERAGE NUMBER OF CHEMICALS: 11
MOST WORRYING: Octinoxate, Isophthalates.
POSSIBLE SIDE-EFFECTS: Allergies; irritation to eyes, nose and throat; hormone disruption, linked to changes in cell structure.

BLUSHER:
CHEMICALS: 16
MOST WORRYING: Ethylparabens, Methylparaben, Propylparaben.
POSSIBLE SIDE-EFFECTS: Rashes; irritation; hormonal disruptions.

FOUNDATION
CHEMICALS: 24
MOST WORRYING: Polymethyl methacrylate.
POSSIBLE SIDE-EFFECTS: Allergies; disrupts immune system; links to cancer.

DEODORANT:
CHEMICALS: 15
MOST WORRYING: Isopropyl Myristate, 'Parfum'.
POSSIBLE SIDE-EFFECTS: Irritation of skin, eyes and lungs; headaches; dizziness; respiratory problems.

BODY LOTION
CHEMICALS: 32
MOST WORRYING: Methylparaben, Propylparaben, Polyethylene Glycol, which is also found in oven cleaners.
POSSIBLE SIDE-EFFECTS: Rashes; irritation; hormonal disruption.

Pesticides, herbicides, GMOs in our food, fluoride and chlorine and trace pharmaceutical residue in the water supplies, methane, carbon monoxide and industrial pollutants in the air, and the toxic chemicals in our everyday household products.

No wonder our bodies are completely bombarded and overwhelmed with the constant exposed to toxic chemicals through the air that we breathe, the water we drink, the foods we eat, and the personal care products and cleaning products we use.

Every Cell in your body responds to the foods you eat, the products you put on your body to the house hold chemicals that you purchase for your home. All of these things have a direct impact on your hormones and in return your hormones have a direct impact on every major system in your body. Not to mention that our body is lacking certain nutrients that heavily influence the function of every cell in our body.

The foods that we consume, oh, the foods we consume.

I haven't used store bought toothpaste in years. I didn't give up brushing my teeth although sometimes I would like to create my very own six foot "personal space bubble." My teeth are beautifully white and my breath is always fresh. After being diagnosed with hypothyroidism, as I continued to research. I was amazed at the things we willingly without even thinking put in or on our bodies that are very harmful to us. I started to take a closer look at all the labels of EVERYTHING and decided that I needed to divorce my store bought toothpaste.

Most of us just focus on diet in an effort to achieve overall better health, along with proper supplements and working out. Oral health is connected with the rest of the body and it's easy to forget where the first step of digestion occurs: Yes, in the mouth!

Why would you continue to use toothpastes that include sodium lauryl phosphate, triclosan, glycerin, fluoride, and other potentially harmful chemicals? Next time you're in the store, take a moment and look at the warning labels on a standard tube of toothpaste or go to your cabinet right now and look at them!

Did you know that your teeth are living and spongy? The foods we eat, the commercial toothpastes, medications and chemicals from drinks all can suck out the minerals from the teeth causing weakened enamel and leaving us more susceptible to decay and breakdown. Being on this new quest for my health I also wanted to keep my teeth healthy by using only the absolute necessary and needed trace minerals to maintain the upmost dental health plus find a solution that wasn't abrasive, while gently polishing them, and detoxifies while it refreshes. Don't I sound like a commercial ad? But was there such a thing? I did know that my long history with Mr. Store bought toothpaste was done. Did you know that there is a tooth paste that could whiten your teeth, remove plaque, and not contain any harmful chemicals or questionable additives?

Sorry, Mr. Toothpaste. I thought we were great together but actually you're slowly killing me. So, it's not me. It's you, and here's why:

Did you know that fluoride was Once Prescribed as an Anti-Thyroid Drug? Up through the 1950s, doctors in Europe and South America prescribed fluoride to reduce thyroid function in patients with over-active thyroids (hyperthyroidism). (Merck Index 1968). If you haven't already, you should invest in a water filtration system to rid your tap water of fluoride. Do you really know how safe tap water is? Look at the recent events in Flint Michigan! Can you really trust the water companies? Although fluoride concentrations in tap water are relatively low and are considered "safe" for human consumption, it is not. Fluoride has long-term neurological and hormonal affects. Fluoride is not an essential nutrient. It is also that chemical that is commonly found in most toothpaste brands. There is clear evidence that, when ingested at high doses, fluoride causes neurotoxicity.

Fluoride also is understood to interfere with the absorption of iodine, possibly leading to an iodine deficiency and ultimately hypothyroidism. To benefit your health, use fluoride free tooth or make your own tooth paste. Get a good water filtration system and purchase a filter for your shower head. We use a British Berkefeld and I also use their brand for a shower filter.

Store bought toothpaste also have other ingredients in it like:

Glycerin is used in almost all toothpastes because it helps create a pasty texture and prevents it from drying out. Although it's non-toxic it coats the teeth just enough to that prevents normal tooth remineralization. Remineralization is a whole-body process and in order for it to happen, the body must have adequate levels of certain nutrients, especially fat soluble vitamins and certain minerals. If you want to stop and reverse Tooth Decay you must add minerals in your diet, add plenty of fat soluble vitamins (A, D, E and K), and your body must be able to absorb vital nutrients. You certainly can't do this by having a coat on your teeth that will prevent absorption.

Sodium Lauryl Sulfate (SLS) is a foaming agent and detergent that is commonly used in toothpaste, shampoo, and other products such as degreaser for car engines. SLS is an estrogen mimicker. It also increases gum inflammation and mouth ulcers. According to a study conducted the Department of Oral Surgery & Oral Medicine in Oslo, Norway, individuals who used a toothpaste containing SLS suffered from more ulcers (canker sores) than those who used an SLS-free toothpaste.

Sweeteners: Sorbitol, sodium saccharin and other artificial sweeteners are often used in toothpaste to improve taste, even though there is no evidence that these sweeteners are beneficial (or even safe) for use in the mouth. Xylitol has shown some positive benefits for oral health in some studies, but it remains a controversial ingredient in toothpaste.

Triclosan: A chemical used in antibacterial soaps and products. Triclosan was recently found to affect proper heart function in a study at University of California Davis and the FDA is currently re-evaluating it for safety in human use.

Let's not forget to mention that many toothpastes also contain artificial colors/dyes or synthetic flavors. I must admit there are several good natural toothpastes out there and I have tried some of them not all but with my tight budget I will make them for pennies on the dollar. My favorite way to brush my teeth is by using tooth powder. Yes, you read this right. Tooth Powder. Here is my recipe that I use. Feel free to adjust the ingredient's based on your own needs. If you have sensitive teeth you might want to skip the baking soda and salt until you can get used to it.

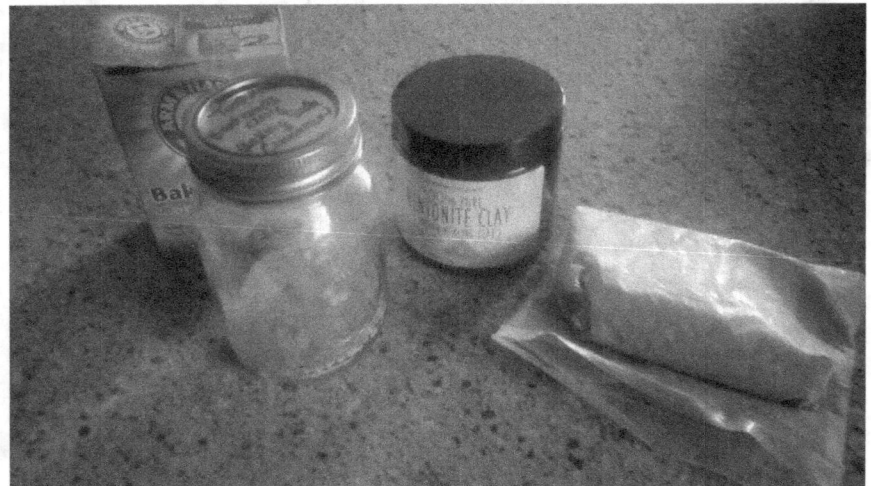

Homemade Tooth Powder Recipe

Ingredients

   4 tablespoons Bentonite Clay

   2 teaspoons baking soda

   1 ½ teaspoons finely ground unrefined sea salt

   ½ teaspoons clove powder

   1 teaspoon ground Ceylon cinnamon

   5-10 drops of peppermint essential oil

   ¾ teaspoons activated charcoal – optional

Directions

Using a stainless steel or plastic spoon, mix all ingredients in a clean glass jar. To use, add a little to a wet toothbrush and brush as normal.

Bentonite Clay

Bentonite clay is a gentle cleanser that is rich in minerals which support tooth remineralization. Its detoxifying properties help freshen breath and fight gum disease, while it's adsorptive properties help remove stains from teeth.

Baking Soda

Baking soda is a mild abrasive tooth polish that helps mechanically remove stains while other ingredients such as clay and activated charcoal draw them out. It also helps freshen breath.

Sea Salt

Unrefined sea salts such as this one contain 60+ trace minerals that aid in tooth remineralization. Salt is also highly antiseptic, which helps keep bacteria in check.

Herb & Spices

Spices and herbs such as clove powder, ground cinnamon, and ground mint add flavoring, but they also have astringent properties that support gum health.

Activated Charcoal

Activated carbon – is made by processing charcoal with oxygen and either calcium chloride or zinc chloride. It was used medicinally by both Hippocrates and the ancient Egyptians, and it is still the poison remedy of choice in modern day emergency rooms. Why? Because it's highly adsorptive, which in plain English means it attracts substances to its surface like a magnet. Like absorptive substances which work like a sponge, adsorptive materials bind with certain compounds and prevent our bodies from using them.

If you're not so hip on using powdered tooth then here are some more all natural recipes.

Natural Tooth Paste Recipe

Natural Peppermint Toothpaste

1/2 cup coconut oil

3 Tablespoons of baking soda

15 drops of peppermint food grade essential oil

Melt to soften the coconut oil. Mix in other ingredients and stir well. Place your mixture into small glass jar. Allow it to cool completely. When ready to use just dip toothbrush in and scrape small amount onto bristles.

Homemade Coconut Oil Toothpaste Recipe

6 tbsp. coconut oil

6 tbsp. baking soda

15-20 drops of a food grade essential oil (peppermint essential oil)

Melt to soften the coconut oil. Mix in other ingredients and stir well. Place your mixture into small glass jar. Allow it to cool completely. When ready to use just dip toothbrush in and scrape small amount onto bristles.

This is a must read powerful book. **The Fluoride Deception** documents a powerful connection between big corporations, the U.S. military, and the historic reassurances of fluoride safety provided by the nation's public health establishment. **The Fluoride Deception** reads like a thriller, but one supported by two hundred pages of source notes, years of investigative reporting, scores of scientist interviews, and archival research in places such as the newly opened files of the Manhattan Project and the Atomic Energy Commission. The book is nothing less than an exhumation of one of the great secret narratives of the industrial era: how a grim workplace poison and the most damaging environmental pollutant of the cold war was added to our drinking water and toothpaste.

FACT: The number of people suffering from hypothyroidism continues to rise each year. Levothyroxine is the 4th highest selling drug in the U.S.

It seems the current medical industry has been abducted by the pharmaceutical industry. In our society we have become so blinded by the Big Pharma propaganda. Once you are labeled with a disease or a condition most of the medications prescribed have horrible side effects and can lead to other issues but in reality these medications only mask the real issue at hand.

"**Our prescription drugs are the third leading cause of death** after heart disease and cancer. Our drugs kill around 200,000 people in America every year, and half of these people die while they do what their doctors told them—so they die because of the side-effects," said Dr. Gotzsche in his recent interview. "The other half die because of errors—and it's often the doctors that make the errors because any drug may come with 20, 30 or 40 warnings, contraindications, precautions and then the patients die."

*NSAIDs as an example of only one group of medications, are fatally toxic to thousands of people each year by damaging joints, lungs, kidneys, eyes, hearts, and intestines and they are covered by insurance companies.

This should come to you as no surprise but some physicians actually receive compensation from the drug industry aka "Big Pharma". (Choudhry, JAMA 2002; 287: 612-617). Also, our part of the government that is in charge of approving drugs called the FDA has advisers with financial ties (and is heavily lobbied by) the very drug industry that is seeking its approval. And as the New England Journal of Medicine and Journal of the American Medical Association warn, even the hired clinical investigators for new drugs may have their price. 'Did you know that 70 percent of Americans are taking prescription drugs?

Even some of our most prestigious journals publish research based on falsified studies, according to Charles Seife, a journalism professor whose class spent a semester trying to figure out why the data doesn't get corrected once research fraud comes to light. "As a result," Seife writes, "Nobody ever finds out which data is bogus, which experiments are tainted, and which drugs might be on the market under false pretenses." **Is Big Pharma America's New Mafia**?

Light Bulb Moment: Why can't we cure what ails us without pharmaceuticals?

Now, if you read anything in this book make sure you hear me when I say," Don't stop taking your medications". Your body may be use to taking these prescriptions and might be dependent upon them. If you decide you want to stop taking them or try to get off your medications. You need to work with a doctor, be monitored and follow their instructions. Your body might need those prescriptions to survive and if you suddenly stop taking them, it might kill you. Therefore, you need to closely work with a Certified Naturopath Doctor or a Knowledgeable Health Practitioner in your area.

Throughout history medical science has sometimes been proven to not be that true in their "research". These words like case studies, credible scientific evidence, scientifically tested, scientific experiments and scientifically proven facts are all merely "theories" until they are proven wrong.

· Bloodletting was once proven to cure most illnesses. Now we all know that it is considered totally ineffective.

· Margarine was considered much healthier than butter. Now new research suggests the complete opposite.

· Eggs were considered very bad because of high cholesterol. Now new research suggests that they are actually healthy for the body.

· Chocolate and oily foods were considered one of the main causes of acne. Now new research suggests that they really don't have an effect on acne.

· Medical doctors said soy based and these added chemicals for baby formula was much better than breast milk for children. Now we know the truth. Breast milk is best.

· Milk was once recommended for coating the stomach and alleviating stomach ulcers. Now it's been discovered to aggravate ulcers.

· Medical science stated that your diet had absolutely no effect on disease or illness. Now we all know diet has a huge effect on the prevention and cause of disease.

· Medical science once had scientific evidence that the removing of tonsils and appendix improved health and should be done to virtually everyone. Now the medical community has reversed that theory.

· Children with asthma were told to stay in enclosed pool areas because the humidity was good for their asthmatic condition. Now new research shows that the chlorine in the air from the pools actually aggravates and makes the asthma worse.

· The most obvious example of all is the fact that there are thousands of drugs that have been approved by the FDA because they were scientifically proven to cure or prevent disease, in addition to having been said to be safe. Now, years later, many lawsuits later, many have been taken off the market because they have been proven that they didn't cure or prevent those diseases. Amongst many who have died or had nearly fatal side effects from the medications.

16 Quotes on medications our doctors prescribe.

1. "The cause of most disease is in the poisonous drugs physicians superstitiously give in order to effect a cure." Charles E. Page, M.D.

2. "The greatest part of all chronic disease is created by the suppression of acute disease by drug poisoning." Henry Lindlahr, M.D.

3. "Every educated physician knows that most diseases are not appreciably helped by medicine." Richard C. Cabot, M.D. (Mass. Gen.Hospital)

4. "Medicines are of subordinate importance because of their very nature they can only work symptomatically." Hans Kusche, M.D.

5. "If all the medicine in the world were thrown into the sea, it would be bad for the fish and good for humanity" O.W. Holmes, (Prof. of Med. Harvard University)

6. "Drug medications consists in employing, as remedies for disease, those things which produce disease in well persons. It is simply a lot of drugs or chemicals or dye-stuffs in a word poisons. All are incompatible with vital matter; all produce disease when brought in contact in any manner with the living; all are poisons." R.T. Trall, M.D., in a two and one half hour lecture to members of congress and the medical profession, delivered at the Smithsonian Institute in Washington D.C.

7. "Drugs never cure disease. They merely hush the voice of nature's protest, and pull down the danger signals she erects along the pathway of transgression. Any poison taken into the system has to be reckoned with later on even though it palliates present symptoms. Pain may disappear, but the patient is left in a worse condition, though unconscious of it at the time." Daniel. H. Kress, M.D.

8. "Every drug increases and complicates the patient's condition." Robert Henderson, M.D.

9. "Medicine is only palliative, for back of disease lies the cause, and this cause no drug can reach." Wier Mitchel, M.D.

10. "The person who takes medicine must recover twice, once from the disease and once from the medicine." William Osler, M.D.

11. "Medical practice has neither philosophy nor common sense to recommend it. In sickness the body is already loaded with impurities. By taking drug – medicines

more impurities are added, thereby the case is further embarrassed and harder to cure." Elmer Lee, M.D., Past Vice President, Academy of Medicine.

12. "Our figures show approximately four and one half million hospital admissions annually due to the adverse reactions to drugs. Further, the average hospital patient has as much as thirty percent chance, depending how long he is in, of doubling his stay due to adverse drug reactions." Milton Silverman, M.D. (Professor of Pharmacology, University of California)

13. "Why would a patient swallow a poison because he is ill, or take that which would make a well man sick." L.F. Kebler, M.D.

14. "What hope is there for medical science to ever become a true science when the entire structure of medical knowledge is built around the idea that there is an entity called disease which can be expelled when the right drug is found?" John H. Tilden, M.D.

15. "The necessity of teaching mankind not to take drugs and medicines, is a duty incumbent upon all who know their uncertainty and injurious effects; and the time is not far distant when the drug system will be abandoned." Charles Armbruster, M. D.

16. "We are prone to thinking of drug abuse in terms of the male population and illicit drugs such as heroin, cocaine, and marijuana. It may surprise you to learn that a greater problem exists with millions of women dependent on legal prescription drugs." Robert Mendelsohn, M.D

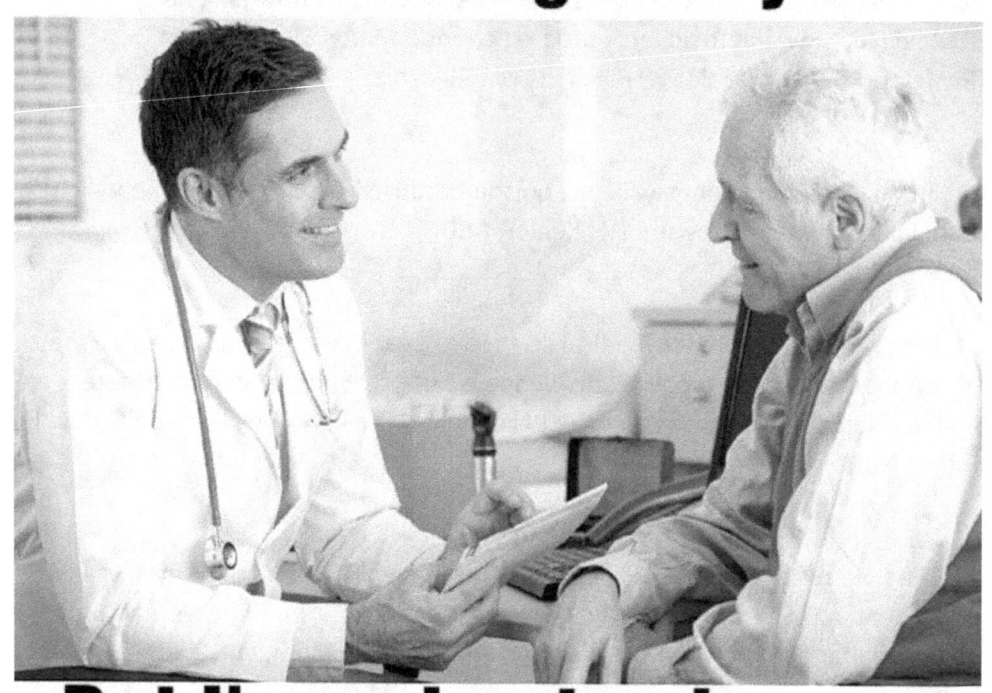

Are you starting to see my point?

The root cause of nearly all diseases can be linked to an overload of toxins and chemicals accumulating inside your body. Most people ignore the toxic overload that is taking a toll on their bodies. Western medicine has taught us that almost all illnesses are caused by germs or genetics. So the money making solution is to slap a name on it. Label each disease (over 10,000 of them) and then have us believe that each one can be remedied by surgery or drugs.

Think about it this– fish can't live in toxic water, no matter how fancy the food is that you're feeding them.

Neither can our bodies thrive if they are toxic.

6 Things you need to working on. I will go into more detail further in the book on each of these 6 things.

#1: Immune System

#2: Digestive System

#3: Inflammation

#4: Stress

#5: Start Being Aware

#6 Rule out other causes of your symptoms

Iron imbalance

Blood sugar imbalances

Nutrient deficiencies

Selenium deficiency

Vitamin D deficiency

Candida Yeast overgrowth

Magnesium deficiency

Digestion issues

Gluten intolerance

Food Allergies

"I don't know where to start"

I know, there is so much information overload that most people are confused as to where to start. You can start by taking ownership of your health. I wanted you to understand or get an idea of how everything has a part to play in your body. I am on a path to help you, lead you and inform you through this terrible illness. Being diagnosed with hypothyroidism isn't just here take this pill and it will fix your issues. Hypothyroidism has a root cause. Once you start addressing the root of your problems then your body can start healing itself. Your body is an awesome design but there is a complex balance between everything. It's a domino effect. If you have something in your body that is overworked it will cause a major shift in your body.

Have you heard of TPO antibodies?

Thyroid peroxidase (TPO), is an enzyme normally found in the thyroid gland, it plays an important role in the production of your thyroid hormones. A TPO test detects antibodies against TPO in the blood. ... In autoimmune disorders, your immune system makes antibodies that mistakenly attack normal tissue.

When you have a higher level of TPO antibodies in your body it may mean that you have Hashimoto's thyroiditis.

You no longer have a "regular" thyroid condition. It's now an autoimmune disease. This "autoimmune disease" has your very own body attacking itself and does its best to destroy your thyroid gland. Your body thinks your thyroid gland is a foreign invader much like a bacteria, virus, fungi, parasites and its going do its best to protect and destroy.

Did you know that your treatment should change if you have thyroid antibodies in your blood which means you have inflammation and your body has an autoimmune disorder. When you lower your inflammation and reduce autoimmunity it will also start to lower your TPO antibodies.

Getting on the right medication to restore your thyroid hormone levels with T4 & T3 are very important but if your TPO antibodies (autoimmune disease) is not addressed, then you're like a hamster on a wheel. Round and round you go don't expect your thyroid hormone to flow.

As a patient with hypothyroidism has your doctor checked to see if you have TPO antibodies? If not, this means many patients with Hashimoto's are being mismanaged and having TPO antibodies changes everything.

The Beginning Factors that start to lead to an Underactive Thyroid

1. Fix your gut!

If you have a leaky gut and you correct this problem by removing the leaky gut trigger foods and start to repair the gut. Now, if you start to heal your gut and your autoimmunity issue isn't normalized then you must continue on your search. Every Cell in your body responds to the foods you consume. These foods have a direct impact on your hormones and in return your hormones have a direct impact on every major system in your body. So many of us have these crazy phantom-like health problems. Our body is lacking certain nutrients that heavily influence the function of every cell in our body while certain foods can inhibit your body's ability to absorb the replacement nutrients needed.

2. Chemical Exposure.

Did you know that products we use every day may contain toxic chemicals and has been linked to women's health issues? They are hidden endocrine disruptors and are very tricky chemicals that play havoc on our bodies. "We are all routinely exposed to endocrine disruptors, and this has the potential to significantly harm the health of our youth," said Renee Sharp, EWG's director of research. "It's important to do what we can to avoid them, but at the same time we can't shop our way out of the problem. We need to have a real chemical policy reform." The longer the length of ingredients on your food label means how much more unhealthy it is for you to consume. When an item contains a host of ingredients that most likely you can't even pronounce or remember to spell you can bet your lucky dollar that the natural nutrients are long gone. These highly processed frank n foods are very difficult for the body to break down and some of the chemicals will become stored in your body. Look at it another way. When is the last time that you see a Azodicarbonamide grazing in a field or Sodium benzoate being grown in a garden?

Environmental chemicals and toxins, pesticides, BPA, thyroid endocrine disruptors, iodine imbalance, other medications, fluoride, overuse of soy products, cigarette smoking, and gluten intolerance. All of these play a very important role in your thyroid health. A nonprofit group called Beyond Pesticides warns that some 60 percent of pesticides used today have been shown to affect the thyroid gland's production of T3 and T4 hormones. Commercially available insecticides and fungicides have also been involved. Even dental x-rays have been linked to an increased risk of thyroid disorders.

3. Go Gluten Free!

You have to start removing the thyroid suppressive foods that are in your diet and instead focus on the right foods that stimulate your thyroid to produce an abundant amount of thyroid hormone to keep your cells happy and healthy. When you eat foods full of thyroid suppressive toxins it's just like throwing fuel on the fire. This will only continue to drain you of your energy, continue to make your symptoms worse, promote even more inflammation in your body, contribute to a leaky gut and further damage your thyroid.

Gluten intolerance is pretty common than previously recognized. It's a major trigger for autoimmune conditions. By removing wheat, barley, and rye products, as well as corn, oats, millet, and coffee you are allowing yourself to heal. You must give it a 3-month try to really see if there's a difference.

4. Start Dry Brushing!

The lymphatic system is responsible for collecting, transporting to the blood, and eliminating the waste our cells produce," "If the lymphatic system is congested, it can lead to a build-up of toxins, causing inflammation and illness. Dry brushing stimulates the lymphatic system as it stimulates and invigorates the skin."

How do dry brush? Start at your feet and brush upward towards the heart. Use firm, small strokes upwards, or work in a circular motion. For the stomach, work in a counterclockwise pattern. Harsh exfoliation is never the point; be sure not to press too hard, or use too-stiff of a brush. "Any kind of brushing or exfoliation should be gentle and should never break the skin."

5. Stress

Stress is one of the worst thyroid offenders, as your thyroid function is intimately tied to your adrenal function, which in turn is intimately affected by how you handle stress.

Many of us are under chronic stress, which results in increased adrenalin and cortisol levels, and elevated cortisol has a negative impact on thyroid function. Thyroid hormone levels drop during stress, while you actually need more thyroid hormones during stressful times.

When stress becomes chronic, the flood of stress chemicals (adrenalin and cortisol) produced by your adrenal glands interferes with thyroid hormones and can contribute to obesity, high blood pressure, high cholesterol, unstable blood sugar, and more. A prolonged stress response can lead to adrenal exhaustion (also known as adrenal fatigue), which is often found alongside thyroid disease

6. Rule out other causes of your symptoms

Iron imbalance

Blood sugar imbalances

Nutrient deficiencies

Selenium deficiency

Vitamin D deficiency

Yeast overgrowth

Magnesium deficiency

Digestion issues

Gluten intolerance

Food Allergies

The most important thyroid nutrients and their doses (for adults) are zinc (30 mg/day), selenium (200 mcg/day), iodine (150 mcg), and iron (18 mg). The uber-cool thyroid pharmacist Izabella Wentz also suggests that low thiamine (vitamin B1) may be an issue for Hashimoto's sufferers, and that supplementing this nutrient may be helpful and a the B-complex.

7. Detox!

You should detox. Why? Well, here is several good reasons. Start removing those toxins from your body and that metal build up. It also gives your immune system a kick start. Its helps to clean out that waste in your digestive tract. It also allows your body to start absorbing nutrients and helps to restore your bodies balance. I've started doing a 16:8 Intermittent Fasting this is basically allow my body to detox daily. I detox for 16 hours and only eat for 8. It also give my digestive system a break and it's not constantly working to break down food.

8. Avoid Tuna, mackerel (King), marlin, orange roughy, shark, swordfish, and tilefish which are the highest in mercury. Heavy metals can bind to your thyroid and thyroid hormone receptors, and interfere with thyroid function.

9. I learned the hard way that not everyone does well on NDT, (aka Armour) some do better on synthetics, especially when they have Hashimoto's. The similarity of pig thyroid to human thyroid can encourage lymphocyte attacks on the thyroid gland.

(This is where my story takes a strange turn of events. I was on Levothryroxine. I am my own health advocate and I am always researching. I asked my doctor to switch me to WP Thyroid. A natural thyroid medication. I couldn't take it. I was sick, gained 15lbs, chest pains and every side effect you can imagine. Then I read up on NP Thyroid. I switched to that. Gained 15 more lbs. and I experienced again every side effect none to man. By this time, I was over it all. I started doing my own "therapy" but I don't recommend that to anyone. This is my body, my life. I started eating like I recommend in this book, intermittent fasting 16:8, if you look back in our history people were doing intermittent fasting before it was in style. I starting making my own cleaning chemicals, reading labels, listening to what my body needed, fake food is the worst thing for your body and if I couldn't eat it, it didn't go on my body. After 2 months of no thyroid medications of any kind and doing it my way. I went back in for blood work. My blood work results came back perfect. I was no longer had hypothyroidism, nor low iron, no more high blood pressure. My doctor suggested that if I still felt sluggish, he would prescribe me a low dose of levoxthryroine. I replied, "No thanks!" I would like to say that I had switched doctors before any of this took place. I am so glad that I did. He had a listening ear.

Not many doctors do. I came in onetime with a written list of things that I needed to cover and wanted to make sure that I wouldn't forget to ask. He took the list from me and went over each thing. One by one and made sure that I felt comfortable before I left with my questions and his answers. Now, this is the 1ˢᵗ doctor since all this began that actually seemed to be alert and again had a "listening ear". Now, let's get back to the journey.)

Consequences of Hypothyroidism- Extreme Exhaustion

People and their doctors sometimes disregard these side effects that come along with hypothyroidism as a natural ageing process. There are close to 300 symptoms that you can experience with hypothyroidism. Many people suffer from fatigue, weight gain, depression and memory loss to just name a few. Some of these symptoms are a side effect as we age, our bodies do start to wear down. You don't have to accept these seemingly "age-related" diminishes as part of your everyday quality of life.

I was always tired, no matter how many hour of sleep I got each night. I had constant brain fog. I was always cold when others weren't. No matter what I did I couldn't shed the lbs. These issues go hand in hand with my diagnosis of hypothyroidism. After being prescribed my hypothyroidism medications I still was having problems. It wasn't getting any better. Many doctors over look adrenal fatigue since it is so similar in comparison with my hypothyroidism. The tests for thyroid and adrenal fatigue are often difficult to understand. The two are often confused or misdiagnosed. So, which one do you treat 1st? The chicken or the egg?

According to the Endocrine Society, adrenal fatigue is a myth promoted by health books and alternative websites. " There is no scientific facts to support the theory that long-term mental, emotional , or physical stress drains the adrenal glands and causes many commons symptoms," the society says on the Hormone health network website.

Symptoms of adrenal fatigue are very similar to symptoms of hypothyroidism. People might experience all of these are just a few. Some of the common ones are:

Trouble concentrating

Find it difficult to obtain quality sleep

Racing thoughts

Decreased sex drive

Body aches

Extremely tired

Moodiness and irritability

Feeling overwhelmed

Hormone imbalance

Cravings for sweet and salty foods

So what can you do about it? Although Extreme Exhaustion is very common with people who have hypothyroidism. There are ways that you can start fighting back.

Start eating foods that help replenish your energy so you can give your system a chance to come back to full health.

Next start removing food that are toxic to your body

Avoid environmental chemicals

Avoid caffeine

Avoid sugars and artificial sweeteners

Avoid microwaved foods

Avoid processed foods

Avoid Hydrogenated oils

Now, you need to start adding nutrient-dense foods that are easy to digest and have beneficial healing qualities. These foods are low in sugar and have healthy fats along with much needed fiber.

Olives

Avocado

Cooked Cruciferous vegetables (Limit this to no more than 2x per week)

Fermented foods

Fatty fish (e.g., wild-caught salmon trout, tuna and mackerel.)

Chicken and Turkey (organic hormone & Antibiotic free)

Grass Fed Beef

Leafy greens

Nitrate free bacon

Nuts, such as walnuts and almonds

Seeds, such as pumpkin, chia and flax

Coconut Flour, Almond Flour and hemp seeds

Chia Seeds

Kelp and seaweed

Celtic or Himalayan sea salt

Low carb fruits and vegetables

Coconut oil

Organic butter (preferably Grass fed)

Ghee

Bone Broth

Eggs: Look for pastured or omega-3 whole eggs

Cheese: Unprocessed cheese (cheddar, goat, cream, blue or mozzarella).

Fish oil (EPA/DHA)

Magnesium

Vitamin B Complex

Vitamin C

Vitamin D3

Zinc

Ancient Nutrition- Bone Broth Collagen Loaded with Bone Broth Co-Factors

Another thing you want to keep in mind is supplementing with the right supplements. Of course, eating the right foods will start to heal your body. It's sad but try most of the fruits and vegetables that we consume don't have the same amount of nutrition as they once did 50 years ago due to soil depletion (from over-farmed and unhealthy farming practices.

Some supplements will help give your body an extra boost. These supplements are:

Magnesium

Fermented fish oil

Ashwagandha

Holy basil

Vitamin B5

Vitamin B12

Vitamin C

Vitamin D3

Zinc

Lastly, you want to start giving you mind and body a rest.

Rest when feel tired.

Sleep 8–10 hours per night.

Avoid staying up late and stay on a regular sleep cycle.

Watch funny movies and laugh with friends

Do something you enjoy daily

Minimize work and relational stress.

Exercise

Avoid negative people and negative self-talk.

D something relaxing

Talk with someone for any traumatic experiences

Find a support partner or group (Our Facebook group Healing Hypothyroidism is a great place to start)

My Chaotic life undiagnosed with Hypothyroidism and Adrenal Fatigue

Being always tired, no matter how many hour of sleep I got each night, was no fun. The constant brain fog and always being cold. No matter what I did that muffin top wasn't coming off. After being prescribed my hypothyroidism medications I still was having problems. It wasn't getting any better. The doctors will tell you to wait 6 weeks and come back for blood work then we can adjust the medication if need be. Many doctors over look adrenal fatigue since it is so similar in comparison with hypothyroidism. The tests for thyroid and adrenal fatigue are often difficult to understand. The two are often confused or misdiagnosed. So, which one do you treat 1st? The chicken or the egg?

What were my adrenals glands?

My adrenals and my thyroid have a strange relationship. They contradict each other all the time. They have a topsy-turvy relationship in which when one thing goes up, the other goes down. My adrenals are my "lifesaving" organs because they control my body's hormones and help me to survive in stressful situations. The adrenals act as the control organs for my "fight or flight" response and secrete many of our most important hormones including: pregnenolone, adrenaline, estrogen, progesterone, testosterone, DHEA and cortisol.

Adrenal fatigue is more often than none misunderstood as an autoimmune disorder. Adrenal fatigue can impersonate and look like other common illnesses and diseases. Adrenal fatigue can be caused by:

Stressful experiences like death of loved one, divorce or surgery

Exposure to environmental toxins and pollution

Prolonged stress due to financial hardship, bad relationships or work environment, and other conditions that entail feelings of despair

Negative thinking and emotional trauma

Lack of sleep

Poor diet and lack of exercise

Unknowingly my adrenals were constantly stressed which set off a chain reaction to my immune system and set up shop for inflammation through my entire body. The adrenal-hypothalamus-pituitary reaction circle controls the release of cortisol. All of my organs and my immunity were being impacted negatively by the resulting continuous hit of cortisol. Actually since my adrenals were out of whack it was causing my hypothyroidism to be much worse than it would be normally. That probably was the reason for my latest diagnosis of Hashimoto's. Could my weakened adrenal glands be the main reason why I developed a thyroid condition in the 1st place? My life was a chaotic world wind of craziness. School fulltime, work fulltime and 3 kids' active children. Does this sound familiar to any of you? Yes, I was exhausted mentally, physically and what was that thing called sleep? Years of poor eating habits and/or chronic stress had finally caught up with me. All those carb loaded, over processed, refined foods and sugars had also caused an imbalance in my insulin and cortisol hormones.

According to the Endocrine Society, adrenal fatigue is a myth promoted by health books and alternative medicine websites. "There are no scientific facts to support the theory that long-term mental, emotional, or physical stress drains the adrenal glands and causes many common symptoms," the society says on the Hormone Health Network website.

The constant abuse that I put on my adrenal glands from the bad eating choices and chronic stress lead to more secretion of cortisol which weaken my adrenal glands and lead to my adrenal fatigue.

Symptoms of adrenal fatigue are very similar to symptoms of hypothyroidism. People might experience all of these are just a few. Some of the more common ones:

- Extremely tired, especially in the morning

- Find it difficult to obtain quality sleep

- Crave sweet and salty foods

- Feel stressed out most of the time

- Decreased sex drive

What I've come to understand is in most cases, a malfunctioning thyroid gland isn't the actual cause of the problem. Hypothyroidism has a root cause. My goal was to figure out what was causing my weakened adrenals and to start addressing those issues. 1st I started to address what I ate. I added more things like:

Olives

Avocado

Cruciferous vegetables (cauliflower, broccoli, Brussels sprouts, etc.)

Fatty fish (e.g., wild-caught salmon)

Chicken and turkey

Nuts, such as walnuts and almonds

Seeds, such as pumpkin, chia and flax

Kelp and seaweed

Celtic or Himalayan sea salt

Coconut

Coconut oil

Organic Kerry Gold butter

Ghee

Fish oil (EPA/DHA)

Magnesium

Vitamin B5

Vitamin B12

Vitamin C

Vitamin D3

Zinc

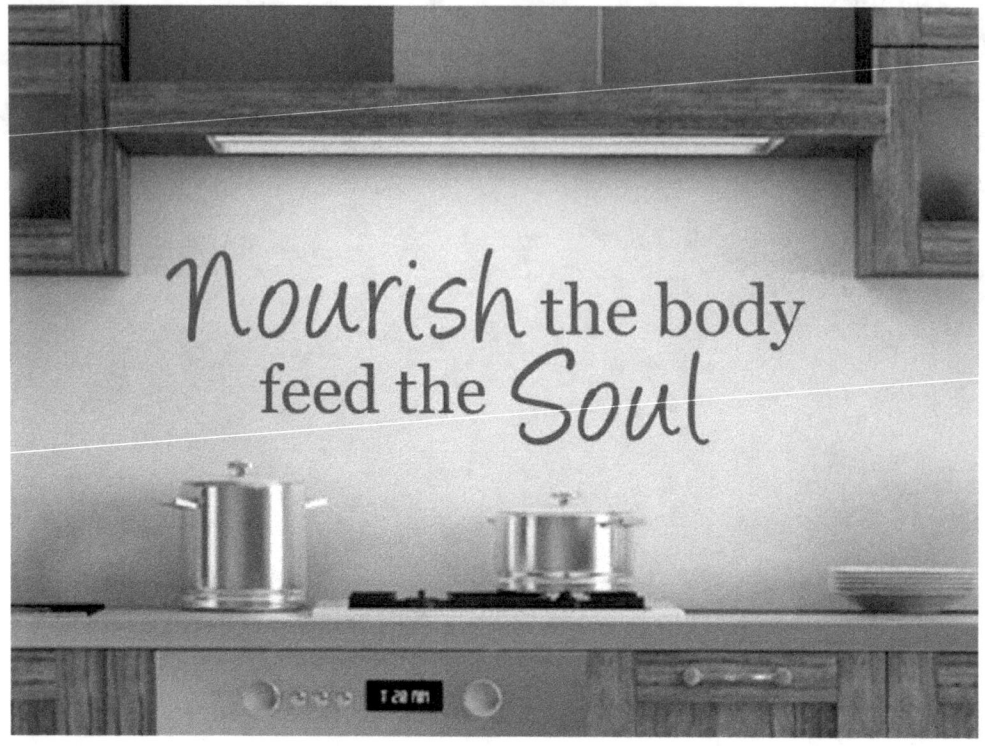

Chapter 2

Cultivating a Healthy Mindset

You know that healthy habits make sense, but did you ever stop to think why you practice them?

I've heard women, in particular, say this a lot lately. They say, "Why can't I look like that?!" I will never look like that!"

Why do we mentally sabotage ourselves? Let's get something clear. You are unique. You are not meant to be me & I am not meant to be you. We are on this planet as individuals, each of us has a unique finger print that can't and won't ever be duplicated with any other human being. Ever! So why do you mentally sabotage your mindset with self-doubt and in return it starts a domino effect on your health? You are telling your subconscious without even realizing it that you are not made for greater things. You are telling your subconscious that you cannot be sexy, be brilliant and be fantastic.

Be happy in your skin.

Everywhere you look — on every billboard, on every social media channel — it seems that there are beautiful, scantily clad women. So it is pushed down our throats that beauty starts from the outside but actually its starts on the inside and radiates outward.

Here's the thing: if you treat your body like it's your worst enemy – or not take ownership of your physical wellbeing – you are repelling good health.   you're keeping yourself from being the best you can be in your life, because you dislike your body so much.

You're basically saying, "I dislike good health. I want to be rid of it."

Well, wish granted!

Good nutrition is an important part of leading a healthy lifestyle

You're meant to make a difference in this world; that's why you're here. But you must believe you're meant for greater things, so you can actually enter a place of mental stability, and eventually, a place of fantastic health. Don't take yourself out of the game by ignoring your bad relationship with your health.

The good you do today, will often be forgotten. Do well anyways. Give the best you have, and it may never be enough but give your best anyways. What you may spend years creating others could destroy it overnight. Keep in mind, it has always been between you and GOD. It was never between you and them anyways.

Try to seek a room full of "different" minded people, for no one grows when they sit in a room full of "like" minded ones! Most people have crippled themselves by their own limitations and try to impose that view on you. You will find that people are often unreasonable, irrational and self-centered.

We all get super busy in this thing called life. Sometimes we lose a little piece of ourselves traveling back in fourth. We can challenge ourselves in small ways that are attainable and be able to stick to these changes in our lives. Trying a new idea each day isn't that difficult. Open up your mind to new possibilities and a new way of being. Honestly, after all, it takes approximately 30 days to break a bad habit and create new more positive change that can last.

Get your mind in a great place first, and it makes everything else much easier.

Each day people will offer you advice and their opinions but what you need to know is they can only understand from the paths that they have walked and their experiences up until that moment. This doesn't make it wrong but you have to listen with open ears.

Life is not a singular vision!

While our ancestors have been around for about six million years, the modern form of humans only evolved about 200,000 years ago. Civilization as we know it is only about 6,000 years old, and industrialization started in the earnest only in the 1800s. Currently there are over 6 billion people on this planet. Everyone who has lived and died have all been unique.

You don't have to repel health. Instead, build your relationship with it.

Investing in myself by joining a group program for a healthier lifestyle is the best thing I ever did for myself. Committing to my personal growth, speaking with people who has been there and done it, and finding the support of like-minded people was crucial to my success and confidence. I've created a group on Facebook called Healing Hypothyroidism? Where you have a "safe place" to share progress and chat with one another.

It's time for you to change your health story and start becoming a healthier you! You can change the game. You can see get a healthier you and change your unhealthy past to make a better future in your life. Make the decision that it will happen for you, and work on your healthy mindset.

Take Action: Create a food journal. Write down everything you eat. Think about what you eat and if it benefits your body. I'm talking old school pen and paper.

Break those chains where you can become a healthier you. Once you see what you eat, you can quickly start to know the area's in your food journal that you need to make a change.

Yes, it can be frightening. It takes a lot of courage to face your unhealthy habits in such detail. Now you can create a health plan to cut unhealthy habits and bring in the health you desire.

1. Improve your relationship your health

When you decide to improve your relationship with your health, be prepared for people to question and criticize you. Change can be a very difficult thing for many of us to handle. You have the mindset, to step out on faith to get the perfect health that you really wish to have. It could be from grabbing that apple instead of those chips, walking 10 minutes per day, or reading a self-help book.

Take Action: Let yourself out of that unhealthy , fast-food, over processed and artificially filled food habit because it's ruining your life.   The only way to create a different outcome is to allow yourself to forgive what's happened in the past. The past does not have to be your future. You are 100% capable of changing your future health story, so do it.

2. You never step outside your box.

"I can't afford eat better."

"I don't want to spend the money on a new lifestyle change book."

"I wish, someone would just give me the magic pill for my ideal body!"

"I don't want to purchase another program that isn't going to work."

Does any of this sound familiar? The more you focus on what you don't have, the less likely it is that you'll ever have it.

Take Action: Focus on what you do haveright now. Express gratitude for literally being alive. Now, you have to create a strategy to have what you really want. Set a goal, writing down realistic goals and make yourself a deadline. Take steps to get there. (And don't quit if it doesn't work the very first try.)

Or... you can keep focusing on what you lack. Call me in a year and tell me how that's working out for you.

3. You think health is something you're granted with, rather than invest.

You want your health to work for you, so you have to think of everything you eat as an investment. Will eating that cheeseburger build or create that healthy body? Probably not.

Will investing in self-improvement books or a mentorship program? Perhaps, if you do the work and commit to changing old habits.

Take Action: When you're about to improve your health, think carefully about why you're about to modify your life with. If that item, service or experience is worth it. Then ask yourself:

Will it feel like a good investment in 90 days, 6 months, or even a year?

Will it help you create a healthier you?

Will it help create a happier you?

Will this change bring you immense joy and memories that will last forever?

Will you grow as a result?

Investing in your health will have a high return, personally and professionally. Don't go foolishly looking for cheap thrills and expect to be in better state of health this time next year. Believe that you're worthy of investing in yourself and believe you'll have a return.

7 Things Women Should Know About Self Image

I've struggled with body imagine my entire life. I was the skinny girl who you seen eating all the time but I could never gain any weight. I had a very high metabolism. After high school started. I was often teased and harassed, and started to become quite self-conscious about being too skinny. The girls would whisper, giggle and call me names.

Of course, we all have that picture perfect imagine that we want to see when we look in the mirror. For some strange reason we think that our lives would be so much easier, if we could just be "that" size. As women, we seem to allow ourselves to be critiqued by the world's view of our self-image and this can affect our self-esteem.

1. Love the Skin Your In

You're the only person in this world that is you. You are unique individuals and that is fantastic. Embrace who you are. You are beautiful. You are worthy. You are enough. Accept yourself and love all your flaws.

2. Find Your Tribe

You are not everyone's cup of tea. We need to feel connected, supported and loved. Finding your tribe of friends will allow you to feel accepted, appreciated and understood. Your tribe will also give you the confidence to stop pretending and be yourself. Keep your standards high, feel good in your own skin and be happy. Soon, you will find yourself surrounded by loving people who will encourage and empower you.

3. Healthy Habits

Good nutrition is an important part of leading a healthy lifestyle. You can do anything that you set your mind to do. Your new healthy habit can be anything from meditation, eating better or trying out a new exercise. Any decision to improve your overall health will benefit you in the long run. Choose a healthy habit that is easy to start. Remember that your life goals isn't your healthy habit change but it will get you started in the right direction. Don't forget this is all a process. Each day you will become better, stronger and more successful.

4. Embrace Life

We live in a fast paced superficial world. Where ever you go, there you are. You can't always control the world around you. Take time to breathe everything in, think about what is going on and let circumstances unfold as they may. Why not allow the universe catch you.

5. Gather Together

I enjoy hanging out with my friends and family over a nice meal. Social connections help us maintain a sense of belonging. Attending a dinner party is heartwarming and it brings people closer. "People with social support have fewer cardiovascular problems and immune problems, and lower levels of cortisol — a stress hormone," says Tasha R. Howe, PhD, associate professor of psychology at Humboldt State University.

6. Think of Others

Volunteering makes a difference in the lives of other people. Studies have shown that people who volunteer and donate their time feel more socially connected. Many people find volunteer work to be helpful with respect to stress reduction, boost your self-confidence and give you a over satisfaction of happiness. A 2012 study in the journal Health Psychology found that participants who volunteered with some regularity lived longer.

7. Gratitude

Gratitude means you're thankful for what you have. You count your blessings by noticing the simple pleasures in life. You also acknowledge everything that you receive. You have learned to live your life as if everything was a miracle, and you are aware of everything that have been given to you. Being thankful changes your mindset from what your life lacks to the abundance that you currently have. One way you can start to practice gratitude daily is by keeping a journal of everything in your life that you are thankful to have. Don't wait for something good to happen to practice gratitude. Start seeing the good in every situation. This will help you improve you self-image. It's not what others think about you, it's what you think about yourself that truly matters.

10 Ways to Deal with Judgmental people

I'm sure you've dealt with judgmental people at some point in your life. You may even feel like you're always dealing with them. It hard to understand sometimes why people think they have an opinion about my life. Why is the world so full of judgmental people? There will always be someone out there judging me no matter what I do.

But here's the thing, it turns out that the people in our lives are reflections of ourselves. Birds of a feather, flock together? See you have to keep in mind that what other people say is not a reflection of you but a reflection of them. This may be hard to swallow at first, but it's true.

I've always had this thrown in my face but understand the concept has taken me well into my 40's and I've finally accepted it. Trust me, it's not easy but it makes sense when you really think about it. When I finally understood this, I realized that I myself was placing a lot of judgment on other people too. What I mean by that is that I often looked at strangers who were doing something different and instantly formed opinions of them in my head, such as "she's crazy, that's not normal behavior, what is she thinking, why is she so weird?" Does this sound familiar? I love to watch people. I can remember sitting on a side bench at Carowind's Amusement Park, waiting for my children while they are in line to get on a ride. Just watching people as they go by. Imaging what they are saying, trying to read their lips and yes, of course throw out judgment.

You might as well admit it, I know for a fact that you've done this too (judging people) because we all do it. The problem is some of us do it a lot more than others. When I realized what I was doing, I felt sort of ashamed and I did not want to be so judgmental anymore, so I made every effort to cut it out. I wanted to try to understand, be more curious, less judgmental. Try to put the shoe on the other foot sort of thing.

Today, I still do catch myself but rarely snap judgments of people and when I do, I think about how I would feel and how I have felt. I try to analyze it, be curious and wonder, "Why"?

If you are finding yourself surrounded by a lot of judgmental people, here are some tips on how to deal with the situation:

1. **Look in the mirror.**

Do you need to sweep your front porch? Many people are so full of themselves. They have so many skeletons in the closet but yet are worried about your pile of trash. But we have to look in the mirror. Not worry about them and ask ourselves, "Why am I being judgmental? Why do I find myself judging people on and what does that have to do with me, what can I work on to better myself?" Think about what areas of your life need improvement and list ways your can begin to heal those areas. You are enough! There is only one you and you are very unique and wonderful. Embellish who you are. Do not undermine your worth by comparing yourself with others.

2. **Practice compassion.**

When you know people are judging you. Try to put yourself in the other person's shoes and realize that they're feeling insecure about themselves for some reason. Something in their life isn't right. They're probably feeling down and disconnected from themselves and don't know how to deal with it. You try to be the better person and treat everyone with love, respect and understanding even if they are criticizing you. Understand that their harsh behavior has nothing to do with you but with the way they feel about themselves. If they are just being assholes tell them to, "Go take a long walk on a short pier". You certainly don't need that negativity in your life.

3. **Look for the lesson.**

Choose to believe that every experience you encounter is trying to teach you something. Get in the habit of finding the lesson you're meant to learn every time someone judges you for something. Thank God when you realize what that lesson is. Instead of getting all bent out of shape, choose to see the deeper meaning behind coming across a harsh person. Be thankful that you are NOT that person. Going through whatever they are going through.

4. **Appreciate the good side of it.**

Instead of getting angry when someone criticized you, appreciate and realize that your message is getting across and people are noticing what you have to say. If you're blogging or writing for example, like me, and you're starting to get some negative feedback, celebrate that you're actually getting through to people and being heard. I'm absolutely ecstatic when I see a comment on one of my threads. Good or bad! I feel that for every negative feedback, I have 10 times more positive feedback (probably even much more), so I don't dwell on the negative, but focus on the positive. Leave me some feedbacks!

5. Accept all feedback.

If you're at all in a public eye of any sort, like I am, be prepared to receive all types of feedback. Especially if you're asking people for their honest opinion, be ready to hear what you don't like. Too often we say to someone, "Be honest, tell me what you really think", but in reality we're not prepared at all to hear anything negative. You have to practice receiving honest feedback and appreciating it for its value. You don't have to always like it, but you should always be open to it objectively. You are valuable. Value yourself enough to walk away from a bad situation, value yourself enough to walk away from a person who doesn't love you the same.

6. Don't take things personally.

If someone you know is judging you harshly, know that it is probably because they judge themselves harshly. Just think," would they kiss their mother with that opinion"? Some people just don't like seeing other people make it. It's that simple. Don't take it personally. Don't make their negativity your own. Don't let their toxic words go to your heart. Don't poison yourself with things that have little or nothing to do with who you are.

"Don't take anything personally. Nothing others do is because of you. What others say and do is a projection of their own reality, their own dream. When you are immune to the opinions and actions of others, you won't be the victim of needless suffering" — Miguel Ruiz

7. Look beyond appearances.

Learn to look beyond appearances, to really see and hear what their soul is saying, not their ego trip, wants you to see and hear.

Look beyond appearances, behind the harsh and toxic words, and see if you can find that place within them where love, beauty and kindness resides. If not, don't let is sit inside you. Let it go. Like a duck allow was to flow off its back. Try to look for the good in people and trust that by doing so you will help bring out the good that lies in them. People won't always see your vision and that is okay. It's your vision not theirs. It's your destiny. Not theirs. Walk your path.

"When another person makes you suffer, it is because he suffers deeply within himself, and his suffering is spilling over. He does not need punishment; he needs help. That's the message he is sending." ~ Thích Nhất Hạnh

8. The world is your mirror

"As a man changes his own nature, so does the attitude of the world change towards him this is the divine mystery supreme. A wonderful thing it is and the source of our happiness. We need not wait to see what others do." ~ Mahatma Gandhi

I have come to realize that whenever I lose control over my thoughts and whenever my thinking isn't that positive and uplifting, that's when things start to go wrong in my world. I'm just in a bad mood. I need to recap, refocus and reenergize.

Like attracts like. If there's darkness within, there will be darkness without. The world is our mirror, it reflects back what's already within us. If the people that come your way are filled with negativity and toxicity and if you feel that you have many interactions of this kind, you might want to start purifying your thoughts and cleansing your own inner world. Get a new porch to sit on, so to speak. What I mean by that is find new friends. Change your circle.

9. Adopt an attitude of gratitude

"I have learned silence from the talkative, toleration from the intolerant, and kindness from the unkind; yet, strange, I am ungrateful to those teachers." ~ Khalil Gibran

Get into the habit of expressing your gratitude and appreciation for every interaction and every experience life sends you way, no matter if good or bad. Use them all to enrich your life and who you are, to grow, to expand and to become the beautiful and wonderful being you were born to be. If you don't appreciate what God has already given you why would he give you more to NOT appreciate.

10. Focus your energy and attention upon those who love and appreciate you

Don't waste your time judging the people who judge you, instead, channel your energy on loving the people who love you. Use your precious time and energy to show your love and appreciation to those who love and adore you.

"When you meet anyone, remember it is a holy encounter. As you see him you will see yourself. As you treat him you will treat yourself. As you think of him you will think of yourself. Never forget this, for in him you will find yourself or lose yourself." ~ A Course In Miracles

Sometimes there are particularly difficult people in our lives or that we come across, and there is absolutely nothing we can do about it. If all else fails, just try to avoid them as much as possible and focus on your own life. You know the old saying," Misery loves company" and trust me. It's true!

Lessons I've learned from Hypothyroidism

Many people don't know about the thyroid and what it does until after they've been diagnosed with hypothyroidism.

1. Thyroid Medication Usually Needs Tweaking

"Many people may feel frustrated when they first start taking replacement thyroid hormones as there can be a lot of trial and error before we get the right dose," says Melanie Goldfarb, MD, director of the Endocrine Tumor Program at John Wayne Cancer Institute at Providence Saint John's Health Center in Santa Monica, California. "It can take three to four weeks for the medication to take effect, and it can take a while to get on the right dose, too."

2. Medication Should Be a Morning Ritual

I've learned to take my medication as soon as I get up along with a warm lemon water with my thyroid medication.

Lemons are loaded with healthy benefits, and particularly, they're a great vitamin C food source. One cup of fresh lemon juice provides 187 percent of your daily recommended serving of vitamin C — take that, oranges! Lemon juice also offers up a healthy serving of potassium, magnesium and copper.

It Aids in digestion and detoxification. It tricks the liver into producing bile, which helps keep food moving through your body and gastrointestinal tract smoothly. Lemon water also helps relieve indigestion or ease an upset stomach.

I've also learned to wait 1 hour before I eat and wait 4 hours before you take any other vitamin supplements because it can interfere with the absorption of your medication. I've also found out that If I wanted to drink coffee I must wait 1 hour after I've taken my medication because it can also interfere with the absorption of your thyroid medication and to never ever to forget to eat breakfast! I need fuel but I have to wait 1 hour after I've taken my thyroid pill.

3. Let thy food be thy medicine

Food is not just calories it is information. It talks to your DNA and tells it what to do. My most powerful tool to change my health was my fork. I needed to stop going long periods of time without food. My body always needed energy. If my blood sugar starts to drop this creates a stress reaction and now your adrenal glands will do what it needs to do to maintain my body's function by releasing more cortisol or adrenaline. Eating often would help put my body back in its normal cycle. I needed to eat foods that nourish my body and not hinder it.

I really had no idea how powerful food really was until after I was diagnosed with Hypothyroidism. Many people with hypothyroidism are deficient in Magnesium, B-12, Zinc, Iodine, B2, Vitamin C, Selenium, Vitamin D and Vitamin A.

The Standard American diet in a nutshell is loaded with unhealthy saturated and trans fats. Our meals are unbalanced, over-sized and loaded with sugar, salt, artificial ingredients and preservatives. We have an abundance of food at our finger tips but yet we are extremely malnourished and mineral deficient. We are literally starving our bodies to death! People are not obtaining the basic nutrients their bodies needs in order to fuel what is needed to perform its proper functions. We are literally running on empty! There is about 20 million estimated Americans with some type of hypothyroid disorder.

Although my thyroid is small, it produces a hormone that influences every cell, tissue and organ in the body. My thyroid determines the rate in which my body produces the energy from nutrients and oxygen. So I need to start eating foods that fed my thyroid. I needed to start nourishing my body back to health with foods that jump kicked my metabolism too.

4. There is no one size fits all diet for Hypothyroidism

I started to research to begin to try to understand that there's really not a one size fits all diet for us with hypothyroidism but there are certain ways we can eat that will certainly help begin the healing process. Diet alone wasn't enough to help my body start fighting this battle that is raging in your body. I needed to start addressing other areas in your life that can cause inflammation like Dietary Allergies, Addressing gut health and avoiding Chemical toxins and endocrine disruptors.

5. I had become my own advocate for my health

After being diagnosed my priorities were made clearer. I had to start listening to my body, stop taking my health for granted and continuing to research to figure out what I needed to do to "fix me". I started making my own cleaning products, lotions and deodorant's. Our skin is the largest organ in our body and it absorbs everything we put on it. Here is a recipe that I make all the time for homemade deodorant.

Homemade Deodorant

1/2 cup baking soda

1/2 cup arrowroot powder or 1/2 cup of cornstarch

5 tablespoon unrefined virgin coconut oil

10 drops of grapefruit essential oil or lavender essential oil

(You can pick your favorite scent. I like lavender or grapefruit.)

Mix baking soda and arrowroot together. Melt your coconut oil in the microwave in a microwave-safe bowl. Mix all ingredients (the baking soda and arrowroot powder) with the oil. Pour into clean small Mason jar. Add your essential oil to the Mason jar; close with the lid. Give it a good shake to combine the essential oil with the other mixture. By doing it this way, you can still use that bowl to eat with. Once you mix that essential oil in the bowl, it can only be used for the purpose of making your deodorant. Everything you've used is edible except the essential oils.

6. **Stop Stressing the Small Stuff**

My thyroid has been having a relationship with my adrenal gland. It's never been straight forward with my body and it never will be. The butterfly shaped gland that sits in front of my neck does more than control my metabolism. My thyroid puts out hormones in my body that knock on every cell and tells it what to do basically but for some reason with my hypothyroidism those cells simply refuse to answer that door.

My adrenal gland is only the size of a walnut and are locked on top of each of your kidneys. She is in charge of producing vital hormones that help regulate your body's functions which include two major important things in your life my sex hormones and my cortisol levels. When you have hypothyroidism your cortisol levels are naturally higher than someone without hypothyroidism. You see I've learned that my Cortisol is more than just a steroid hormone that is made in the cortex of the adrenal gland. It has a greater task than just being tagged as your fight or flight response system. Almost every cell in my body contains receptors for cortisol. When my stress levels are high cortisol is released into my blood stream. Our bodies aren't designed for us to be in a constant state of emergency. Our adrenal glands doesn't know the difference between a true emergency and just being stressed out. So in return she will continue to produce extra cortisol into our blood stream. After a while of pumping out the constant need for cortisol she will become weakened and start decreasing her ability to produce cortisol and instead produce extra adrenaline. So do you see why we must get our stress under control and not stress the small stuff! Let things roll off our back like a duck does water.

7. Start Addressing the Root Cause of my Hypothyroidism

I needed to understand or get an idea of how everything has a part to play in my body. Being diagnosed with hypothyroidism wasn't just here take this pill and it will fix my issues. Hypothyroidism had a root cause. Once I started addressing the root of your problems then my body can start healing itself. My body is an awesome design but there is a complex balance between everything. It's a domino effect. If I had something in my body that is overworked it can cause a major shift in my body. Two things I needed to start doing immediately is getting my immune system in check and decreasing inflammation. Inflammation disrupts the production and regulatory mechanisms of thyroid hormones. Sometimes we have to do a little pruning of the branches, in order for the tree to be healthy again. A number of things can be the reason why I had hypothyroidism. It could be a wide range of things from celiac disease, Hashimoto's, leaky gut, autoimmune disease disorder, nutrient deficiency's, adrenal fatigue, exposure to chemicals, gluten or other food allergies, and hormonal imbalance. It most defiantly started with the foods that I was eating and the chemicals in the environment, my thyroid could be influenced by many different circumstances. I needed to start figuring out what the root cause of my hypothyroidism was.

8. Start Loving Myself Again

All I do is run, run and run! I am exhausted and felt so guilty anytime I needed to have down time because there was things that needed to be done. So I started to allow myself to take a day and do nothing. I mean absolutely nothing. WHY? Because my body needed to recharge and stop being ran into the freaking ground. I am not a machine. I started taking Epsom salt baths. I will also take a day where I lay around and watch movies. Get up take a shower and put on more pajamas.

We all have to die someday but do me a favor. Don't die not trying, don't die not seeking after the truth, don't die just accepting this is your fate. It's up to you to make a difference in your life. This your life, your body and your choice. We all have a story. You are the author of your book, make it fantastic. In my book: A Survivors Cookbook Guide to Kicking Hypothyroidisms Booty. I have over 200 recipes that show you how to start fighting hypothyroidism with your fork.

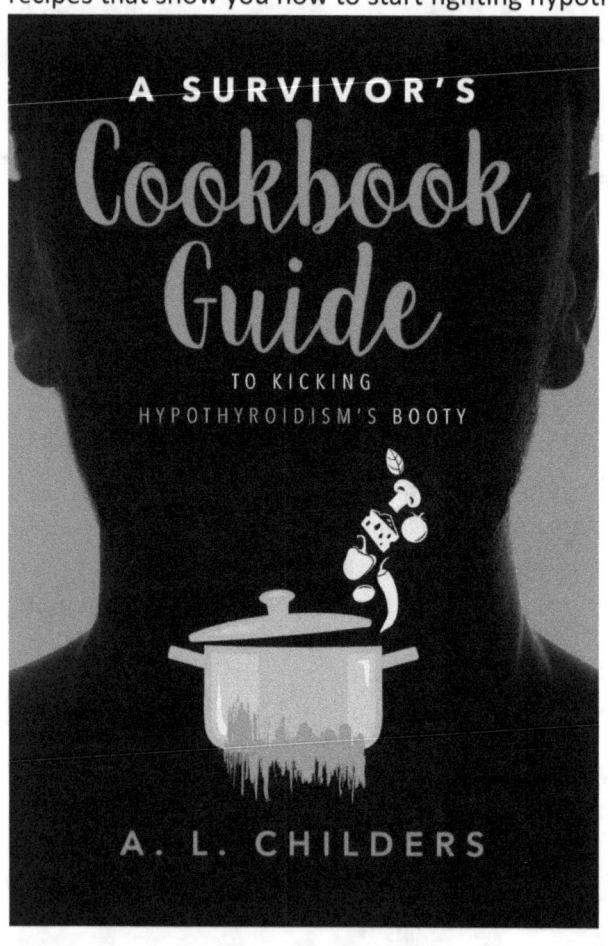

Chapter 3

Chronic Candida Attacking Your Thyroid?

Our lives already seem to be on hold from our hypothyroidism. Did you know that an overload of Candida was picked up at birth or shortly thereafter? We were supposed to be getting good friendly bacteria from our mother's at birth, but "our" mothers could have had a Candida overgrowth and unknowingly passed it on to us. And over the years, our bodies has become more and more compromised. Your gut microbes could be dramatically affecting your thyroid health. There is a lot of misinformation and misunderstanding about Candida. Both from the medical profession and on the internet. It is easy to get fooled into thinking, as many sites will try to convince you, that all anyone need to do is to take their product or buy their e-book. Of course, they will all have testimonies. What these testimonies fail to mention is if you continue on the path your on and don't change the Candida comes back — maybe in a month or two or in six months. It just depends on however long again it took for the Candida to overgrow enough to start causing symptoms. . It is important to know that dealing with Candida is not an easy fix.

"Hypothyroidism causes low body temps which allows fungal overgrowth. Get the temps up and the fungal/yeast will have nowhere to live."

The first antibiotic, penicillin, was discovered by Alexander Fleming in 1928. The use back then was pretty small compared to how they are used now for everything!! These antibiotics work on killing the bad bacteria but also in the process killing your good bacteria. In the 1950's Sugar and refined carbohydrate consumption surged. All these refined carbohydrates reduces your good bacteria and creates an imbalance where candida can flourish. Let's not forget that sugar also weakens your immune system, and with a weakened immune system it fight Candida like it should be able to. New exposures to drugs, birth control pills, vaccines, pesticides, herbicides, chemicals, antibiotics are fed in huge quantities to cattle, meat, dairy we consume and chickens we eat. All of this ultimately destroys much of the friendly flora and weakens the immune system so that the oxygen-loving Candida yeast begin to flourish and overgrow in our intestinal tract. A few more things can upset the balance of gut microbes and contribute to yeast overgrowth. Chronic stress, Diabetes, Pregnancy, Eating too many refined carbs, (Sugar is the main fuel for yeast) antibiotics, environmental toxins, birth control pills and steroids.

Side Note: Another thing that is rarely mentioned is parasites. People can have parasites. Don't be alarmed it does happen and if you start to eat this way that I am mentioned below it will help rid your body of them. You can always be tested but that does require a stool sample for your doctor.

Instead of asking for anti-fungal drugs why not give your body a fighting chance. Stop eating that a high sugar and a high carbohydrate diet. If you really want to get rid of the yeast. Remember yeast loves sugar.

Now, you need to start adding nutrient-dense foods that are easy to digest and have beneficial healing qualities. These foods are low in sugar and have healthy fats along with much needed fiber.

Olives

Avocado

Cooked Cruciferous vegetables (Limit this to no more than 2x per week)

Fermented foods

Fatty fish (e.g., wild-caught salmon trout, tuna and mackerel.)

Chicken and Turkey (organic hormone & Antibiotic free)

Grass Fed Beef

Leafy greens

Nitrate free bacon

Nuts, such as walnuts and almonds

Seeds, such as pumpkin, chia and flax

Coconut Flour, Almond Flour and hemp seeds

Chia Seeds

Kelp and seaweed

Celtic or Himalayan sea salt

Low carb fruits and vegetables

Coconut oil

Olive oil

Organic butter (preferably Grass fed)

Ghee

Bone Broth

Eggs: Look for pastured or omega-3 whole eggs (unless you have a food allergy)

Cheese: Unprocessed cheese (cheddar, goat, mozzarella).

Garlic

Onions

Ginger

Lemon/limes

Cayenne Pepper

Fish oil (EPA/DHA)

Magnesium

Vitamin B Complex

Vitamin C

Vitamin D3

Zinc

A high quality multi vitamin like Garden of life

Coenzyme Q10

Ancient Nutrition- Bone Broth Collagen Loaded with Bone Broth Co-Factors

Avoid all forms of sugar like honey, molasses, maple syrup, agave, xylitol, and artificial sweeteners, like aspartame, Splenda.

(Which we will get into later why you should avoid artificial sweeteners!)

No dried fruits or fruit juices.

Check to see if you have a food allergy. The most common ones are gluten, dairy, egg, soy, corn.

Epson salt baths are especially helpful for the yeast die-off symptoms and it's an excellent way to get magnesium for your thyroid! Use 2-3 cups of salt in warm bath and soak 20min.

Start taking a quality probiotic. I take raw probiotics by Garden of Life.

Ginger tea

Ingredients:

1 square inch piece of fresh Ginger root

Squeeze of lemon

2 cup of water

Cut off the outside of the ginger root, then grate it and add to boiling water. Boil for 20 minutes. Strain and serve with a slice of lemon.

Yeast and Parasite Cleanse Drink

10 gloves of garlic, peeled

½ cup of warm coconut oil

1 cup of organic apple cider vinegar

2-inch piece of fresh ginger, peeled

1 tablespoon of Ceylon cinnamon

2 lemons, washed and cut

Blend, strain through a mess strainer, and store in a mason jar in the refrigeration. Put 1 tablespoons in a glass of water on an empty stomach daily. Garlic, ginger, and even lemon can interact with certain medications. Please check with your health care provider to make sure that you won't have any adverse medication reactions if you plan on taking this as a drink with other medications.

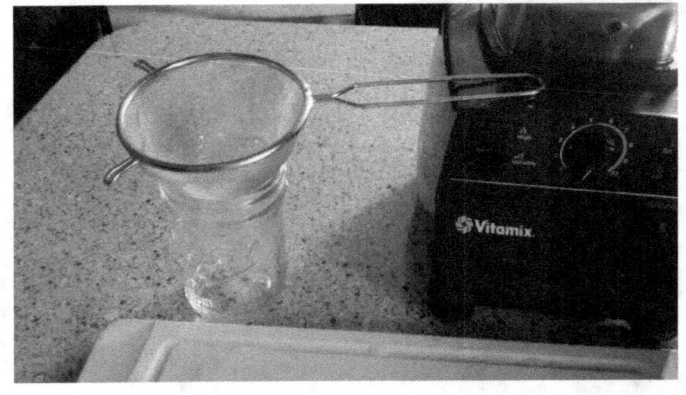

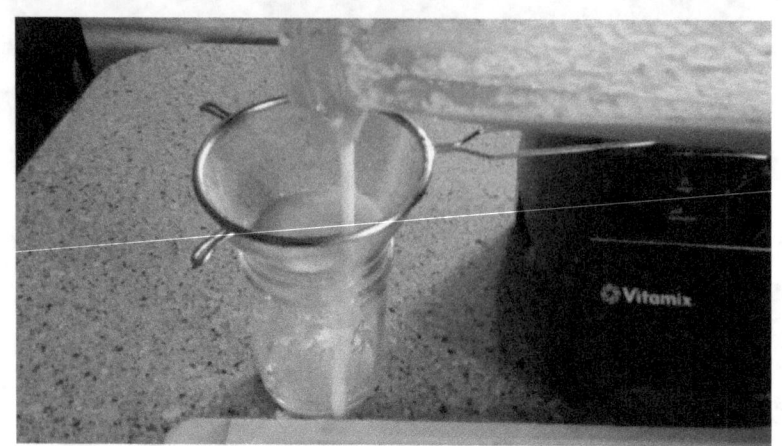

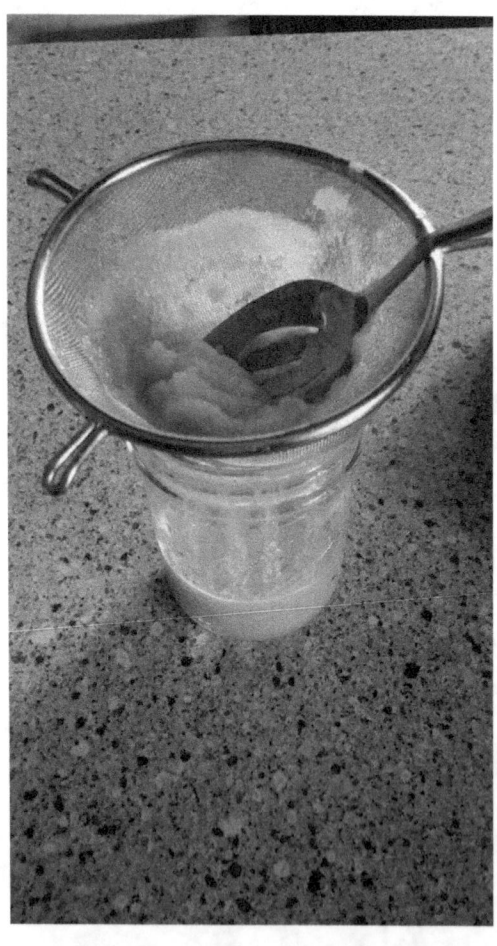

Boosting your Immunity with Better Gut Health

We are creating a perfect storm within our bodies. The less nutrients we consume, more toxins we add, create this world win of health issues. It's sad that our western diet is made up of red meats, vegetable oils, white flour and sugar. Who would have thought that something so simple as eating has become so complicated?

Food does matter. It talks to your DNA. Food can change your DNA!

The foods you eat have a major impact on autoimmune disease — It affects your gut health and along with increasing or decreasing the inflammation in your body. Unfortunately, our western world diet are full of foods that have a bad impact on both your gut and your inflammation. Start with eating whole foods that are anti-inflammatory. For instance, omega-3 wild fish, leafy greens and turmeric. If it was made in a lab, avoid it. Do a little research and you will find that our western diet that is made up of processed, fake foods, chemicals, sugar and corn oils are all highly flaming the fan of your inflammation. Begin to start reading labels. You will soon discover that health foods such as low-fat and gluten-free packaged foods, which are often loaded with sugar, additives, and preservatives. Grains, dairy, legumes, eggs, corn, and soy are not the cornerstones to a healthy diet anymore they can contribute to a leaky gut and inflammation. Did you know that Gluten triggers the release of a chemical called zonulin, which tells the walls of your intestines to open up and by doing so this releases toxins into your bloodstream.

Feed the masses and feed them cheap

Think about what you're putting in your body. Either you're fighting disease or feeding disease. You must get a concept of nutrient density. Many of the foods we tend to eat, block nutrients from being absorbed. Gluten, dairy and soy products create inflammation in the digestive tract. In ancient times grains were prepared by **soaking, sprouting and fermenting** but that tradition in making them been long forgotten with our fast-paced culture. If you have inflammation in the digestive system undigested proteins leak into the blood stream creating a heightened immune reaction that often makes your thyroid issues worse and can lead to a leaky gut which causes other problems.

Your gut is your portal to health. It houses 80 percent of your immune system, and without your gut being healthy it is practically impossible to have a healthy immune system. A leaky gut have been linked to hormonal imbalances, autoimmune diseases such as rheumatoid arthritis and hashimotos thyroiditis, diabetes, chronic fatigue, fibromyalgia, anxiety, depression, eczema and rosacea, and that is just to name a few. So you can understand why a properly working digestive system (your gut) is vital to your health.

Contrary to what we use to believe. We now know that having a leaky gut is one of the main reasons, and probably the beginning stage, for developing an autoimmune disease. Having a leaky gut means that the tight junctions that usually hold the walls of your intestines together have become loose, allowing undigested food particles, microbes, toxins, and more to leave your gut and enter your bloodstream. This will cause your body to become full of inflammation, which in return will start to trigger a autoimmune condition and if you already have an autoimmune condition it will certainly make it worse.

Luckily for you. Your gut is made up of wonderful cells that can turn over very quickly, so you can start to heal your gut in as little as thirty days, by following these 4 R guidelines: Remove, Restore, Replace and Repair

Remove the damage — Remove these inflammatory foods, household & body chemicals, drink filtered water(to avoid fluoride and chloride) , stop using aluminum brand deodorant, start using fluoride free brand tooth pastes, start to reduce your stress that damage your gut, do a detox to heal any gut infections from yeast, parasites, or bacteria.

Restore the Strong — Replenish the enzymes and digestive acids that are necessary for proper digestion

Replace with friendly Bacteria — Make sure you are taking plenty a good strong probiotic that is full of these much needed "good bacteria" to start supporting your immune system. Here is a great product that I use. You can do your own research and I am sure there are other brands out there that are wonderful too. Garden Of Life Dr. Formulated Probiotics Once Daily Women's, 30 Count

Repair the digestive Tract — Give you gut a fighting chance by supplying the nutrients and amino acids needed to build a healthy gut lining. (Gelatin can improve your ability to produce adequate gastric acid secretions that are needed for proper digestion and nutrient absorption. Glycine from gelatin is important for restoring a healthy mucosal lining in the stomach and facilitating with the balance of digestive enzymes (I use   Garden of Life RAW Enzymes Women, 90 Capsules) and stomach acid. The best way to consume gelatin make them into broth or soup. You can do this by simply brewing some bone broth at home using this Bone Broth Recipe. If the appeal of drinking broth from dead animal bones doesn't seem that appealing in-which I personally find the average commercial brand of collagen pretty gross. Most collagen supplements are produced from the bones, skin, and connective tissue of animals, including cattle, fish, horses, pigs, or rabbits. The idea of drinking bones+ connective tissue from dead animals doesn't appeal to me at all. Even if they say it's from "grass-fed animals". YUCK!I I get my COLLAGEN that is made from fish the brand I use is a Marine based Collagen and it is sourced from the scales of wild-caught, non-GMO Red Snapper , wild-caught in the Pacific Ocean near Hawaii using sustainable harvesting instead of being sourced from the hides of pasture-raised, grass-fed bovine.

Probiotics

For most people, taking a quality probiotic supplement doesn't have any side effects other than higher energy and better digestive health. As a society we have drastically cut back on our consumption of vegetables and of beneficial essential fatty acids (flax, pumpkin, black current seed oil, dark green leafy vegetables, hemp, chia seeds, fish) such as those found in certain fish (including salmon, mackerel, and herring) and flaxseed. We are consumed with little fiber and an excess of sugar, salt, and processed foods. Stress, changes in the diet, contaminated food, chlorinated water, and numerous other factors can also alter the bacterial flora in the intestinal tract. When you treat the whole person instead of just treating a disease or symptom, an imbalance in the intestinal tract stands out like an elephant in the room. So to play it safe, I recommend taking a probiotic supplement every.

Probiotics are live bacteria and yeasts that are good for your health, especially your digestive system. Probiotics are often called "good" or "helpful" bacteria because they help keep your gut healthy. Probiotics foods include yogurt, kefir, Kimchi, Sour Pickles (brined in water and sea salt instead of vinegar) Pickle juice is rich in electrolytes, and has been shown to help relieve exercise-induced muscle cramps., Kombucha, kombucha tea ,Fermented meat, fish, and eggs.

Fixing that unhappy belly by providing the nutrients and amino acids needed to start building a healthy gut lining. Most people simply do not understand how complex the human gastrointestinal system is, and contrary to popular belief, your gut isn't just a food processing and storage depot. Did you know that your gut has so much influence on your health is because it is home to roughly 100,000,000,000,000 (100 trillion) bacteria (approximately 3 pounds worth) that line your intestinal tract. Your gut is the home control center to your digestive system, your nervous system, as well as your immune system.

Our digestive system doesn't absorb food, it absorbs nutrients.

My 3 favorite gut healing smoothies!

1/2 – 1 cup unsweetened almond milk

1/4 teaspoon (100 billion units) probiotic

1 scoop (5000 mg) L-Glutamine

1/2 avocado (throw away the seed)

2 Thumb size pieces of ginger, chopped finely and peeled

1/2 teaspoon of flaxseeds or chia seeds

1 teaspoon of raw organic unfiltered local honey

2-4 fresh mint leaves (depending on taste, optional)

1/2 cup frozen organic berry mix (raspberries or blueberries)

1 serving of collagen protein

Blend in a blender and add ice if you like. You can also make this the night before, stick it in a jar and blend it the next morning.

My 3 favorite gut healing smoothies!

1 Banana

1 cup unsweetened Almond milk

1/4 cup gluten-free oats

1 tbsp. Turmeric and sprinkle of black pepper, ground

1 tsp Chia seeds or flaxseeds

1/4 teaspoon (100 billion units) probiotic

1 serving of collagen protein

1 tbsp. Almond nut butter

2 Thumb size pieces of ginger, chopped finely and peeled

Blend in a blender and add ice if you like. You can also make this the night before, stick it in a jar and blend it the next morning.

My 3 favorite gut healing smoothies!

1 cup of coconut milk

1 banana

1/2 cup of mango

1/2 tsp turmeric powder

1/2 teaspoon of Ceylon cinnamon

2 Thumb size pieces of ginger, chopped finely and peeled

1 teaspoon of chia seeds or flaxseeds

1/4 teaspoon (100 billion units) probiotic

1 serving of collagen protein

Blend in a blender and add ice if you like. You can also make this the night before, stick it in a jar and blend it the next morning.

Vitamins and supplements should I be taking for my Thyroid

Vitamins and other nutrients can help fight inflammation, the autoimmune processes and help improve a dysfunctional thyroid but if you don't know what you're needing to supplement they can alter the level of thyroid hormones in your blood and can mask other issues at hand. Supplements can contain various amounts of active ingredients and how do you know what your body needs? Your doctor should perform a series of blood tests to see if your body is deficient. If your doctor isn't really interested in performing these much needed tests then switch doctors find a Certified Naturopath Doctor or a Knowledgeable Health Practitioner in your area.

The Council for Responsible Nutrition, a trade association that represents the dietary supplement industry, acknowledges that thyroid supplements can interact with prescription medications.

When you take your morning thyroid medication. Take it with a glass of freshly squeezed lemon water and no other medications. Wait 1 hour before you eat and then 4 hours before you take any other supplements. Your supplements can interfere with your thyroid medication. If you drink lemon water it helps detox and gets the digestive juices flowing.

Sales of supplements in the United States reached $11.5 billion dollars in 2012.

Sales of all dietary supplements in the United States totaled an estimated $36.7 billion in 2014.

We all know that I am not a doctor but I am a life hacker and a health journalist trying to research and get the word out on the ridiculously overcrowded industry full of shady marketing and dubious claims that are being made.

How can the FDA protect the consumers when it doesn't have a strong history of enforcing the law?

Over a hundred million people taking dietary supplements each day. How can we determine what is safe?

Am I saying that all supplements are bad?

NO, Not at all!

Absolutely most of the supplements being sold are a waste of money. Although, there are situations in which having a supplement IN ADDITION to a quality nutritious diet is very beneficial.

You must read the ingredients! I am currently taking all Garden Of Life Products. No, I don't have an endorsement deal with them but that would be so nice since I only purchase their products. I find their products are high quality, made from plants, no fillers or binders, gluten free and no extra chemicals.

How do I know what supplements to take for my hypothyroidism? Remember there are no shortcuts in reaching your health and fitness goals.

Did you know that there was a massive study and it was determined that for a huge majority of healthy individuals who had no deficiencies what so ever but yet they felt as if they had to take unnecessary vitamins. In fact the vitamins that they were taking were doing more damage than good because it was full of fillers, binders and all was made in a lab. This is where you doctor comes into play. You need to get routine blood work to see if you are lacking anything.

I believe that your main focus should still be on eating a high quality, nutritious diet with plenty of vegetables, and working alongside a doctor they can tell you exactly what your body is missing and from there they can help fill in any deficiencies you may have.

"Are ALL supplements the same?"

Have you read any articles lately on FAKE supplements being sold at Walmart, GNC, and others? The question to ask is, "Are ALL supplements the same?" Absolutely NOT! The kind of vitamin supplement or nutritional supplement that a woman needs depends solely her on own body needs. We all are unique and what I may need your body may not. Another thing to think about some supplements you can find on the shelves contain herbs or other unnecessary ingredients that can be potentially harmful. People can easy overdose on certain nutrients and in large amounts can be very toxic to your health.

It is always best to get your vitamins (as well as minerals) naturally from foods.

Did you know that a 100 grams of spinach has healthy amounts of vitamins A, C, E, K, several B vitamins, and essential minerals including iron and calcium?

Natural vs. Synthetic Vitamins – What's the Big Difference?

Vitamins are little organic molecules we need, certain ones our bodies just can't make and we must rely on our food to keep us stocked with these essential nutrients, but our food is getting less and less nutritious. Fields are depleted by overuse. Pesticides limit the action of beneficial microbes in the soil that help plants draw in nutrients. Fertilizers focus on certain key chemicals that deplete the must needed trace minerals, organic components and the beneficial microbes that go into the good nutrition source of the plant. Then, there are these genetically modified foods have made their way into our food supply.

In this modern age, we seem to have taken steps back instead of forward. Refining and processing our food so it lasts longer, it certainly makes it more convenient and they add chemicals to make it taste better. We've stripped out and destroy the vital nutrients as we process them. Much of the food we find in grocery stores outside the produce section barely resembles what humanity has been eating for thousands of years. These food like substances are at the core of many auto-immune disorders, food allergies, and the growing epidemics of obesity. Our bodies don't know what we're ingesting, they aren't finding the nutrients they need, and our bodies are begging for us to eat more and more so we might manage to give ourselves what we're missing.

Our digestive system doesn't absorb food, it absorbs nutrients.

We all know we need a steady supply of vitamins and minerals so our bodies can function properly. Scientists, doctors, and food companies agree too, so they create cheap vitamins in labs, fortify our foods and beverages with them, and dump them into multivitamins. The problem is these synthetic vitamins are not what our bodies are looking for either.

Almost all multivitamins are from synthetics. The same goes for fortified foods. There's a good reason for this. Synthetic vitamins are cheaper to make and usually more stable. This means they can last on shelves for months or years, be added to foods in high doses, and create small dense tablets packed with insane amounts of every type of vitamin. These vitamins are allowed to call themselves "natural" even when they are actually synthetic because scientists say the synthetics are virtually identical to the ones found in food.

We know that vitamins and minerals are essential for life, and vitamin deficiencies can definitely hurt you. Always read your labels and stay clear of supplements that contain artificial colorings, sodium benzoate, propylene glycol, aluminum silicate and High fructose corn syrup.

So what vitamins and supplements should I be taking to naturally give my Thyroid that needed boost?

So there are **Fourteen nutrients** required for your thyroid to get from your brain creating TSH and stimulating your thyroid gland to produce T4 to T3 and then to activate your cellular metabolic rate. The **Fourteen nutrients** are:

1. Protein

We want to control blood sugar swings this will help us with a healthy thyroid. Eating consistent eating throughout the day of high-quality protein at every meal without eating too many carbohydrates. Remember that blood sugar swings not only affect the thyroid gland itself but also indirectly affect adrenal gland function. You don't always have to eat meat for protein! Lentils, chickpeas, green peas, quinoa, oatmeal, wild rice, chia seeds, nuts, nut butters, broccoli, spinach, asparagus, artichokes, potatoes, sweet potatoes and Brussels sprouts. Remember not all protein is created equal.

I read an article on WebMD, which stated approximately .36 grams of protein per pound of body weight is enough. I weigh 150 pounds, so my intake should be around 54 grams of protein per day. Too much protein is a bad thing. A high-protein diet may backfire for people at risk for heart disease — increasing the likelihood of weight gain and early death, a new study suggests.

2. Magnesium

Magnesium helps you to make more T4 in the thyroid gland. It converts the inactive T4 thyroid hormone into the active form of T3. This is extremely important because the metabolism of your body cells are enhanced by T3, not inactive T4.

Magnesium-rich foods which include almonds, pumpkin seeds, chard, spinach, avocado, figs, and even dark chocolate.

Go with a Magnesium Glycinate brand is a good, it's highly absorbable, this is recommended for anyone with a known magnesium deficiency and less likely to cause laxative effects than some other magnesium supplements. Daily dose of 400 mg no more than 800 mg

3. Zinc

Zinc helps to convert the thyroid hormone T4 to T3. Food sources of zinc include shellfish, mollusks, meat, legumes, and nuts. "If you opt for a zinc supplement, 30 milligrams is sufficient.

Foods high in Zinc are:

Shrimp.

Kidney beans.

Flax Seeds.

Pumpkin Seeds.

Oysters.

Watermelon seeds.

Recommended Daily Allowances. Adult men and adolescent boys between 14 and 18 years of age should aim to consume about 11 milligrams of zinc daily, while adult women 19 years old and over need about 8 milligrams. Girls between 14 and 18 require 9 mg per day.

4. Iodine

We need only 150 mcg of iodine per day in our diet, according to the Institute of Medicine. "That tiny amount of iodine enables the thyroid to manufacture just the right amount of the thyroid hormone thyroxine. Good food sources include milk, cheese, poultry, eggs, kelp, and other seaweeds. "But you have to be careful with supplementing iodine because too much can be problematic and actually cause hyperthyroidism," Keep an eye on your iodine intake. Most people get enough iodine from their regular diet.

5. Vitamin C

This vitamin C helps to reduce adrenal stress. It is also an antioxidant that will reduce "oxidative stress placed on the gland either by foreign toxins and harmful free radicals".

Foods that provide vitamin C are chili peppers, bell peppers, pineapple, mango kiwi, papaya, Brussels sprouts

For adults, the recommended dietary reference intake for vitamin C is 65 to 90 milligrams (mg) a day, and the upper limit is 2,000 mg a day. Although too much dietary vitamin C is unlikely to be harmful, mega doses of vitamin C supplements may cause: Diarrhea. Nausea.

6. Selenium

Selenium supports efficient thyroid synthesis and metabolism. Foods that provide selenium include tuna, shrimp, salmon, sardines, scallops, lamb, chicken, beef, turkey, eggs, and shitake mushrooms. You can also eat 2 Brazilian nuts per day and get your RDA!

Most people can get their RDA of selenium from food. In studies to determine if selenium could aid in prostate cancer prevention, men took 200 micrograms daily. The safe upper limit for selenium is 400 micrograms a day in adults. Anything above that is considered an overdose.

7. Vitamin D

This vitamin helps to transport thyroid hormone in to cells and helps to heal autoimmune thyroid disease. 20 minutes of sunlight a day is a natural way to get free vitamin d.

Foods that provide vitamin D include:

Fatty fish, like tuna, mackerel, and salmon.

Foods fortified with vitamin D, like some dairy products, orange juice, soy milk, and cereals.

Beef liver.

Cheese.

Egg yolks.

Vitamin D intake is recommended at 400–800 IU/day, or 10–20 micrograms. However, some studies suggest that a higher daily intake of 1000–4000 IU (25–100 micrograms) is needed to maintain optimal blood levels.

8. Vitamin A

This vitamin acts on the cells of the body like a hormone because it directly affects the DNA of the cell nucleus directing cellular protein production. The best sources of Vitamin A would be Fermented Cod Liver Oil.

High vitamin A foods include sweet potatoes, carrots, dark leafy greens, winter squashes, lettuce, dried apricots, cantaloupe, bell peppers, fish, liver, and tropical fruits.

Vitamin A is included in most multivitamins, and the U.S. recommended dietary allowance (RDA) for adults is as follows: 900 micrograms daily (3,000 IU) for men and 700 micrograms daily (2,300 IU) for women; for pregnant women 19 years old and older, 770 micrograms daily (2,600 IU); and for lactating women 19 years old.

Other nutrients that are very important to your thyroid health are:

9. Glutathione

Glutathione is a strong antioxidant that helps balance hormones and boost the immune system. Dr. Axe has written an article, 9 ways to boost glutathione, check it out.

10. Probiotics

Probiotics are important to your gut health.

11. Vitamin B Complex

Make sure it has all the b vitamins in it. This vitamin have many interactions with thyroid function and hormone regulation. Good food sources of vitamin B include whole grains, legumes, nuts, milk, yogurt, meat, fish, eggs, seeds, and dark leafy greens.

Recommended dietary amounts (RDAs) are 2.4 micrograms daily for ages 14 years and older, 2.6 micrograms daily for pregnant females, and 2.8 micrograms daily for breastfeeding females. Those over 50 years of age should meet the RDA by eating foods reinforced with B12 or by taking a vitamin B12 supplement.

12. Vitamin E

A contains carotenes which is what the thyroid needs to help it function normally. However, when you take your vitamin E it is also recommended that you have your selenium at the same time as vitamin E because the vitamin can cause an increase in the metabolism of selenium.

Vitamin E Rich Foods List

1) Almonds. 1 oz: 7.3 mg (27% DV)

2) Spinach. 1 bunch: 6.9 mg (26% DV)

3) Sweet Potato. 1 Tbsp: 4.2 mg (15% DV)

4) Avocado. 1 whole: 2.7 mg (10% DV)

5) Wheat germ. 1 ounce: 4.5 mg (17% DV)

6) Sunflower seeds. 2 Tbsp: 4.2 mg (15% DV)

7) Palm Oil. 1 Tbsp: 2.2 mg (11% DV)

8) Butternut squash.

For adults older than 18 years, pregnant women, and breastfeeding women, the maximum dose is 1,000 milligrams daily (or 1,500 IU). For age-related macular degeneration, 30 milligrams to 500-600 IU of vitamin E (alpha-tocopherol) has been taken by mouth daily for 4-8 years.

13. Flaxseed oil

Omega-3 fatty acids can help "decrease inflammation and help with immunity" for thyroid support. Some studies have indicated that omega-3 fatty acids can increase thyroid hormone uptake.

14. Curcumin-

Also known as turmeric. Turmeric can be helpful in reducing whole body inflammation, healing the gut, as well as detoxifying from heavy metals in those with autoimmunity.

Instead of taking all these different supplements undividedly. You can get most of yours from a simple multivitamin but again you really need to get your doctor do perform blood work to see if your lacking anything. As you have read, I am a big fan of Garden of Products but that isn't saying that there aren't other brands just as good but my research lead me to Garden Of Life.

Supplement Ingredients to Avoid

This was in one of my thyroid support pills. I started to have more heart palpitations and my blood pressure was rising. Research- research-and research! Never take anyone word for granted. You must figure out what is best for your body and most important listen to your body.

L-tyrosine- The body naturally produces thyroid hormones. Tyrosine might increase how much thyroid hormone the body produces. Taking tyrosine with thyroid hormone pills might cause there to be too much thyroid hormone. This could increase the effects and side effects of thyroid hormones. It also can block other medications along with interacting. It is possible to end up with hyperthyroidism (overactive thyroid) from supplementing with L-tyrosine.

Kelp, a type of seaweed that is often marketed for thyroid health, is loaded with iodine. For example, a serving (one drop) of Liquid Kelp, a dietary supplement promoted for "Thyroid Gland Support," contains 800 mcg of iodine. "Most people get enough iodine from their regular diet," But if you take a supplement that contains kelp, plus a multivitamin, such as GNC Women's Ultra Mega One Daily containing 150 mcg of iodine, and also use iodized salt that contains 400 mcg of iodine per teaspoon, it's easy to consume far more iodine than your thyroid needs—and that's not healthy for you.

Other tips!

1. Sleep-I try to get at-least 8 hours of sleep per night.

2. Detox baths and wraps

3. Yoga and meditation for relaxation

4. Rebounding to get the body flowing

5. Walking and weight training- are low-impact exercises that can get the heart pumping.

6. Eat more Organic foods which contain fewer amounts of chemicals and pesticides which, as you know from everything so far that I've written in this book that they are thyroid-disrupting chemicals and will have a negative effect on the thyroid gland.

7. If you're needing an awesome cookbook to get you started on healthy eating try my book: A Survivors Cookbook Guide to Kicking Hypothyroidism Booty. It has a ton of recipes in it to get you going!

Remember, there is no one size fits all program when you are dealing with your body. When you start to eat smarter and are aware of what foods feed your body, despite the condition, you can start to feel better and manage your health better. In this age of overly processed, genetically modified, artificially flavored and preservative loaded foods.

The best patient to be is a well informed and an educated patient. My blogs and books can make the difference between you having the energy to live your life as you want, or merely dragging yourself through life.

Here is what a typical day looks like for me. Now you might not need all of this nutrients but I do.

A.M.

Breakfast

Thyroid medication with 24oz of lemon water

Dry Brushing

 Listen up my fellow ladies: The benefits of dry skin brushing are freaking fabulous! It Increases the circulation to the skin and reduced the appearance of cellulite. Helps your skin to absorb nutrients by eliminating clogged pores, boost circulation, stimulate the lymph nodes and improve digestion.

Jump on my rebounder for 45 minutes

Rebounding is a super gentle exercise that reduces your body fat; firms your legs, thighs, abdomen, arms, and hips; increases your agility; and improves your sense of balance. It will strengthen your overall muscles and provide an easy aerobic effect on your heart. Along with having excellent detox and immune building benefits it helps the lymphatic system get rid of that metabolic garbage build up which can be dead and cancerous cells, nitrogenous wastes, infectious viruses and heavy metals. With all this being said why are you not rebounding?

Wait 1 hour eat an approved breakfast from my book

A Survivors Cookbook Guide to Kicking Hypothyroidism Booty

Before I brush my teeth a few times a week I coconut oil pull

I also make my own dry tooth paste the recipe is in this book but if you don't want to do that you can order dirty Mouth or research and find a brand that works for you.

Lunch

Smoothie

1 scoop of Garden of Life Fit

8oz of unsweetened almond milk

2 organic celery stalks

1 small piece of ginger

1/2 cucumber

Handful of organic romaine lettuce

I also add in my vitamins to the mix (yes, I put this in my smoothie since I can't swallow pills)

Vitamin B Complex

Garden of life Multivitamin

Curcumin

COQ10

Probiotics

Odorless Garlic (I pinch a small opening & squeeze it in, discard the shell)

I wait 2 hours then take my iron supplement

Get in 24oz of more water

Somewhere in my day I try to soak up 20 minutes of sun

Snack is normally a Fit Bar by Garden Of life

Dinner

I eat an approved Dinner from my book

A Survivors Cookbook Guide to Kicking Hypothyroidism Booty

Along with My Vitamin C

A few times a week I also have a detox bath or a body wrap

I make sure I get all my water in I have to have no less than 75oz's per day.

How you calculate your water intake is your weight divided by 2

So if you weigh 150lbs divide that by 2 and its 75. 75oz's

Never-ever drink your water intake @ 1 time. People have died from that. Water toxicity.

Not every night but if I feel like it 1-2 glasses of red wine or a Tito's vodka tonic with lime Twist.

Is Your Thyroid Causing Your Digestive Problems?

I've struggled with constipation, diarrhea, bloated stomach or just stomach pain in general. I later found out that it was related to my thyroid. In fact, my thyroid was the root cause for all current health issues.

I had to start removing the thyroid suppressive foods that were in my diet and instead focus on the right foods that stimulated my thyroid to produce an abundant amount of thyroid hormone to keep my cells happy and healthy. When I ate foods full of thyroid suppressive toxins it's just like throwing fuel on the fire. This only continued to drain me of my energy, continue to make my symptoms worse, promote even more inflammation in my body and also contributed to a leaky gut that further damaged my thyroid.

Listen to me when I say there's a major disconnect between what YOU believe to be healthy foods and what research tells us is healthy. In fact, many of the health foods today that people go out of their way to eat daily are extremely thyroid suppressive.

It seems that the testing for thyroid is a dead end road at times with the test appearing to be normal but you has all the symptoms. Get this, your blood work can look just fine but there is major resistance at the receptor site. Most practitioners are unfamiliar with natural treatments for the thyroid and the medications they prescribe sometimes just don't work. Some doctors just don't have a lot of experience with alternative treatments. Endocrinologists have the training to diagnose and treat hormone imbalances and problems by helping to restore the normal balance of hormones in the body. This is where you come into play. You have to take control of your health! Your gut's ability to digest and absorb critical nutrients is very important for proper thyroid hormone health.

There is only one major disease and that is malnutrition. All Ailments and afflictions to which we may fall heir are directly traceable to this major disease."
—D.W. Cavanaugh, M.D., Cornell University

Let me say this again: Hypothyroidism has a root cause. Once you start addressing the root of your problems then your body can start healing itself. Your body is an awesome design but there is a complex balance between everything. It's a domino effect. If you have something in your body that is overworked it will cause a major shift in your body. Don't worry the good news is it can be put in remission.

Food is not just calories it is information. It talks to your DNA and tells it what to do. Your most powerful tool to change your health is your fork. You can't go long periods without food. Your body always needs energy. If your blood sugar starts to drop this creates a stress reaction and now your adrenal glands will do what it needs to do to maintain your body's function by releasing more cortisol or adrenaline. Eating often will help put your body back in its normal cycle. You should eat foods that nourish your body and not hinder it.

Beneficial bacteria supports your immune system

So here we are talking about gut health again! I wonder why this keeps coming back as a discussion.

For most people, taking a quality probiotic supplement doesn't have any side effects other than higher energy and better digestive health. As a society we have drastically cut back on our consumption of vegetables and of beneficial essential fatty acids (flax, pumpkin, black current seed oil, dark green leafy vegetables, hemp, chia seeds, fish) such as those found in certain fish (including salmon, mackerel, and herring) and flaxseed. We are consumed with little fiber and an excess of sugar, salt, and processed foods. Stress, changes in the diet, contaminated food, chlorinated water, and numerous other factors can also alter the bacterial flora in the intestinal tract. When you treat the whole person instead of just treating a disease or symptom, an imbalance in the intestinal tract stands out like an elephant in the room. So to play it safe, again, I recommend taking a probiotic supplement every.

Probiotics are live bacteria and yeasts that are good for your health, especially your digestive system. Probiotics are often called "good" or "helpful" bacteria because they help keep your gut healthy. Probiotics foods include yogurt, kefir, Kimchi, Sour Pickles (brined in water and sea salt instead of vinegar) Pickle juice is rich in electrolytes, and has been shown to help relieve exercise-induced muscle cramps.

Prebiotics foods are brown rice, oatmeal, flax, chia, asparagus, Raw Jerusalem artichokes, leeks, artichokes, garlic, carrots, peas, beans, onions, chicory, jicama, tomatoes, frozen bananas, cherries, apples, pears, oranges, strawberries, cranberries, kiwi, and berries are good sources. Nuts are also a prebiotic source.

The ideal pH for the colon is very slightly acidic, in the 6.7–6.9 range. When there is an imbalance or lack of beneficial bacteria in the colon, the pH is typically more alkaline, around 7.5 or higher. The optimal pH range for gas-producing organisms is slightly alkaline at 7.2–7.3.

When someone starts taking a probiotic or a prebiotic supplement (or eats a prebiotic food), the beneficial microorganisms begin to increase in number. These good bacteria start to ferment more soluble fiber into beneficial products like butyric acid, acetic acid, lactic acid, and propionic acid. These acids provide energy, improve mineral, vitamin, and fat absorption, and help prevent inflammation and cancer. The extra acid also starts to lower the pH in the colon.

You gut is just one of the gateways to your health. If you have developed a leaky gut it means the tight junctions that usually hold the walls of your intestines together have become loose, allowing undigested food particles, microbes, toxins, and more to escape your gut and enter your bloodstream, causing a huge rise in inflammation that triggers or can even worsen any autoimmune condition. Don't worry my friend, you can start to heal your gut in a little as thirty days by incorporating a few easy steps in your life.

Say goodbye to inflammatory foods, toxins, and stress that damage your gut, as well as gut infections from yeast, parasites, or bacteria.

What do you need to do and how do I do start? Eat more plant-based, whole, nutrient-dense foods.

Cut out refined sugar and flour, processed junk and animal products. Start adding a variety of organic plant-based whole foods to your diet. These foods will start to fill your body with the vitamins, minerals, cancer-fighting phytochemicals, antioxidants, and fiber it needs to recover from chronic inflammation.

Say hello to good enzymes and acids necessary for proper digestion.

What do you need to do and how do I do start? Remove grains aka GLUTEN and legumes. Start eating pineapple and papaya. **Our digestive system doesn't absorb food, it absorbs nutrients**. If we don't have enough digestive enzymes, we can't break down our food—which means even if we are eating well, we aren't absorbing all that beneficial nutrition. Have you taken the time to glance at your poop? Here are a few signs that you might need to take a quality digestive enzyme supplement 30 minutes before a meal and make sure it doesn't contain products like gluten, dairy, etc. If it doesn't say "contains no: sugar, salt, wheat, gluten, soy, milk, egg, shellfish or preservatives then avoid them. Read labels! Make sure it has at least these three things in the supplement proteases (which break down proteins), lipases (which break down fats), and carbohydrase's (such as amylase, which break down carbohydrates).

If you have:

Gas and bloating after meals

The sensation that you have food sitting in your stomach (a rock in your gut)

Feeling full after eating a few bites of food

Undigested food in your stool*

Floating stools (an occasional floating piece is fine, but if all your poop consistently floats, that might be a sign something is wrong)

An "oil slick" in the toilet bowl (undigested fat)

Start taking a quality probiotic. By adding in good Bacteria back it will start supporting your immune system and allow your body is get back into balance and flush things out of our system.

Foods like raw garlic, turmeric, Fermented Foods, raw coconut oil, artichokes, onions, asparagus and leafy greens.

I really enjoy eating a raw Golden Beets with Carrot & Ginger. It's organic, raw, fermented and an all-natural quality Probiotic health food.

Fixing that unhappy belly by providing the nutrients and amino acids needed to start building a healthy gut lining. Most people simply do not understand how complex the human gastrointestinal system is, and contrary to popular belief, your gut isn't just a food processing and storage depot. Did you know that your gut has so much influence on your health is because it is home to roughly 100,000,000,000,000 (100 trillion) bacteria (approximately 3 pounds worth) that line your intestinal tract. Your gut is the home control center to your digestive system, your nervous system, as well as your immune system.

Here are two great products that I use. You can do your own research and I am sure there are other brands out there that are wonderful too.

Garden Of Life Dr. Formulated Probiotics Once Daily Women's, 30 Count

Garden of Life RAW Enzymes Women, 90 Capsules

The Role of Food in Your Hypothyroidism Journey

The true role the food industry has in your journey.

In this book, I've hit many areas on why you may have hypothyroidism and it does have a root cause. Now, that you're searching for answers and looking for what could be the underlying reason why you have hypothyroidism, let's start talking more about food.

Many different underlying reasons can play a role. We do know that hypothyroidism is a chronic condition of an underactive thyroid and affects millions of Americans. I've covered how Environmental chemicals and toxins, pesticides, BPA, thyroid endocrine disruptors, iodine imbalance, other medications, fluoride, overuse of soy products, cigarette smoking, and gluten intolerance. All of these play a very important role in your thyroid health.

If you are still unsure what Hypothyroidism means what exactly?

Hypothyroidism means your thyroid is not making enough thyroid hormone. Your thyroid is a butterfly-shaped gland in the front of your throat. It makes the hormones that control the way your body uses energy. Basically, our thyroid hormone tells all the cells in our bodies how busy they should be. Our bodies will go into overdrive with too much thyroid hormone (hyperthyroidism) and our bodies slow down with too little thyroid hormone (hypothyroidism). The most common causes of hypothyroidism worldwide is dietary and environmental. The most common cause of hypothyroidism is dietary and environmental! What does that mean exactly? That means you need to be eat to cater to your thyroid and stop using all these harmful chemicals to clean your home with and put on your body! It's not hard. Yes, a little adjustment will be needed but isn't everything we do in life for the better of our health worth a little inconvenience until it becomes a habit?

"You must realize that the thyroid has a relationship with all the hormones. It's a very complex balance and there is no straight forward treatment of just treating your thyroid alone. 1st you must make sure your adrenal glands are in total support. Adrenal fatigue is a very common amongst people with hypothyroidism. Next you have to get your cortisol levels stabilized. Having hypothyroidism your cortisol levels are already above average. Next finding the right medication for you. Everyone is different it isn't an easy one size fits all task."

One cannot think well, love well, and sleep well if one has not dined well.

—Virginia Woolf 1882-1941, A Room of One's Own

A diet for hypothyroidism should include whole foods rich in iodine:

whole baked organic potatoes with skin, cod, dried seaweed, shrimp, Himalayan crystal salt, baked turkey breast, dried prunes, navy beans, tuna, boiled eggs, lobster, cranberries, and green beans. Niacin-rich foods (required for normal manufacture of thyroid hormone) are tuna, chicken, prunes, bananas, turkey, salmon, sardines, and brown rice.

Riboflavin-rich foods:

Raw almonds, eggs, mushrooms, sesame seeds, salmon, and tuna.

Zinc: (as well as vitamins B6, C, and E, iodine) is a major component of thyroid hormone balance and is antimicrobial. Zinc-rich foods (boost thyroid function) are white cooked button mushrooms, chickpeas, kidney beans, dark chocolate (70 percent or higher), pumpkin, squash seeds, and almonds.

Selenium-rich foods: (helps to convert T-4 to T-3) are Brazil nuts and tuna.

High-polyphenols foods: (acts as an anti-fungal) are cocoa powder, dark chocolate, coffee, tea, flaxseed meal, red raspberries, blueberries, black currants.

Vitamin B6–rich foods: (required for normal manufacture of thyroid hormone) are raw unsalted sunflower seeds, quinoa, raw pumpkin seeds, sesame seeds, flaxseeds, pistachio nuts, cashews, tuna, halibut, salmon, dried prunes, bananas, avocados, dried apricots, and raisins.

Vitamin C–rich foods: (boost thyroid gland function) are bell peppers, dark leafy greens, kiwis, broccoli, berries, citrus fruits, tomatoes, peas, and papayas.

Riboflavin-rich foods: (or vitamin b2—essential for normal manufacture of thyroid hormone) are frozen peas, beets, crimini mushrooms, eggs, asparagus, almonds, and turkey.

Vitamin E–rich foods: (work with zinc and vitamin A to produce thyroid hormone) are raw almonds, shrimp, avocados, quinoa, salmon, extra-virgin olive oil, and cooked butternut squash.

Fatty fish like wild salmon, trout, halibut, cod, albacore tuna, flounder, cod or sardines (omega-3s and selenium) only a few times per week....

No farmed fish, period! Also, with the radiation from Fukushima nuclear meltdown finally reaching our shores in America. I wouldn't eat any kind of seafood.

No gluten.

Split peas, lentils, black beans, kidney beans, pinto beans, artichokes, raspberries, blackberries, chia seeds, red apples with skin, prunes, green peas, raw almonds, garbanzo beans, winter squash, spaghetti squash, summer squash, butternut squash, zucchini, popcorn (no microwave-ready, bagged popcorn), cherries, citrus fruits, kiwi, cantaloupe, papaya, mango, plums and red grapes, tomatoes, carrots, gluten-free, steel-cut oats or gluten-free rolled oats, watermelon, green tea, organic apple cider vinegar, lemon, garlic, leeks, parsley, celery, ginger root, tomatoes, cucumbers, carrots, asparagus, organic whole baked potatoes with skin, shrimp, Himalayan crystal salt, Celtic sea salt, baked turkey breast, dried prunes, navy beans, gluten free steel cut or rolled oats, cranberries and green beans, organic no hormone chicken, brown rice, raw almonds, eggs, sesame seeds, chickpeas, kidney beans, dark chocolate 70 percent or higher, walnuts, cocoa powder, hempseeds, red raspberries, blueberries, black currants, brazil nuts, raw unsalted sunflower seeds, quinoa, raw pumpkin seeds, sesame seeds, flaxseeds, pistachio nuts, cashews, dried prunes, bananas, avocados, dried apricots, and raisins, red, green and orange bell peppers, romaine lettuce, kiwis, papayas, beets, all mushrooms, quinoa, extra-virgin olive oil and cooked butter nut squash. sea vegetables, dried seaweed, kelp, dulse, nori, arame, wakame, kombu, tomato paste, brewer's yeast, brown rice, algae, healing spices (Ceylon cinnamon, turmeric, gloves, cayenne pepper, garlic, oregano, sage, ginger .

See you are NOT limited to what you can eat with hypothyroidism. You have many options to what you can eat and why you need to be eating this. I want you to see what an abundance of foods that you can eat. The only limit you have in the kitchen is your imagination. You can start to creating your favorite recipes and healing your thyroid as you eat! What and how you eat is part of the solution.

This is my list that I stick to. This is what my body needs. I find that it's easier for my body to digest this list that is below. These foods are low in sugar and have healthy fats along with much needed fiber. Now, you see you are not limited and there are many options with abundance of choice. You have no excuse to not start eating nutrient dense foods. Of course, eating the right foods will start to heal your body. It's sad but most of the fruits and vegetables that we consume don't have the same amount of nutrition as they once did 50 years ago due to soil depletion from over-farmed and unhealthy farming practices.

Olives

Avocado

Cooked Cruciferous vegetables (Limit this to no more than 2x per week)

Fermented foods

Fatty fish (e.g., wild-caught salmon trout, tuna and mackerel.)

Chicken and Turkey (organic hormone & Antibiotic free)

Grass Fed Beef

Leafy greens

Nitrate free bacon

Nuts, such as walnuts and almonds

Seeds, such as pumpkin, chia and flax

Coconut Flour, Almond Flour and hemp seeds

Chia Seeds

Kelp and seaweed

Celtic or Himalayan sea salt

Low carb fruits and vegetables

Coconut oil

Organic butter (preferably Grass fed)

Ghee

Bone Broth

Eggs: Look for pastured or omega-3 whole eggs

Cheese: Unprocessed cheese (cheddar, goat, cream, blue or mozzarella).

Fish oil (EPA/DHA)

Magnesium

Vitamin B Complex

Vitamin C

Vitamin D3

Zinc

Ancient Nutrition- Bone Broth Collagen Loaded with Bone Broth Co-Factors

7 Worst Foods for Your Hypothyroidism

So, by now you understand that the thyroid gland sits on the front of your neck and produces a hormone that impacts EVERY SINGLE CELL, TISSUE, and ORGAN in your entire body. How does it do this? The thyroid gland is responsible for maintaining your body temperature, heart rate, and controlling your metabolism. The thyroid gland is very sensitive, meaning that too much thyroid stimulating hormone (TSH) and too little TSH can cause detrimental effects throughout your body. You see, the hypothalamus in your brain (a very small gland that is a BIG deal) produces thyroid releasing hormone (or TRH). {When functioning properly, your thyroid gland and hypothalamus become a feedback loop that constantly keep your thyroid levels in "balance." Think of it as a checks and balances system.} TRH stimulates the pituitary gland to release TSH. TSH stimulates the thyroid gland to actually release the actual thyroid hormones (T3 & T4). T3 & T4 levels are monitored by the pituitary gland which (based upon the amount in free circulation in the bloodstream) either increases or decreases your TRH. And the cycle continues.

So, what happens in those with hypothyroidism? Hypothyroidism is defined as underactive or a low amount of free circulating thyroid hormone (T3 & T4). When the hypothalamus releases TRH, the pituitary stimulates TSH, and T3 & T4 are released. When a person has hypothyroidism, their TSH levels will be elevated but their T3 & T4 levels will be low. These low levels will feed back to the pituitary gland, which will increase TRH, which will increase TSH, and the cycle continues. The brain (hypothalamus that releases TRH) interprets the low levels of T3 & T4 and tries to increase them by increasing TRH and TSH. After all the research I've done I have found that these 7 foods are the worst for my thyroid and I avoid them like the black plague.

#1 Broccoli (And other cruciferous vegetables)

Kale, broccoli and other cruciferous vegetables like cauliflower, and cabbage are not actually "bad" for the thyroid – but if you have hypothyroidism or a goiter it should be limited unless it's thoroughly cooked. "Goitrogen's", can actually prevent your thyroid from getting the iodine it needs to run properly. You thyroid needs iodine to be able to convert it into hormones. Iodine is a necessity for healthy thyroid function. If your iodine is low cruciferous veggies will contribute to your thyroid problems. But you can eat all the fermented cruciferous vegetables and it has no bad effects on your thyroid and it's excellent for your gut health.

The same is true for other cruciferous vegetables like:

Cabbage

Cauliflower

Broccoli

Brussels sprouts

Bok choy

Radishes

Mustard greens

Chard

As you know, these vegetables are excellent in fighting cancer and has many other health benefits so perhaps another solution could be to eat more iodine rich foods along with your cruciferous veggies.

#2 Strawberries (And other fruits containing thiourea)

Strawberries and peaches are "mildly goitrogenic" foods and they contain thiourea.

These fruits carry the compound called thiourea, which poses the same problem as the cruciferous vegetables. As mentioned in #1, "Goitrogen's", can actually prevent your thyroid from getting the iodine it needs to run properly. You thyroid needs iodine to be able to convert it into hormones. Iodine is a necessity for healthy thyroid function. If your iodine is low cruciferous veggies will contribute to your thyroid problems.

Other fruits that contain thiourea are:

Peaches

Pears

Rutabaga

#3 Soy

Brilliant marketing campaigns have lead you to believe that soy products are healthy but in fact it's completely the opposite. Soy products are not healthy foods. Eating soy frequently can potentially lead to numerous other health issues.

For centuries, Asian people have been consuming fermented soy products such as natto, tempeh, and soy sauce, and enjoying the health benefits. Fermented soy does not wreak havoc on your body like unfermented soy products do.

The issue with soy is most soy today contains something called phytoestrogens, and these phytoestrogens are estrogen mimickers in the body. And so, if you're a male consuming extra estrogen, it's going to give you more feminine characteristics.

If you're a woman consuming foods that increase estrogen levels, it's going to increase your risk of breast cancer, cervical cancer, PCOS (polycystic ovary syndrome) and other hormone imbalance-related disorders.

Many have felt as if they needed a diary substitute since they couldn't tolerate dairy. Actually your body was doing you an even bigger favor.

For starters, some chemicals such as isoflavones, found in soy products like soy milk or edamame, can intercept your thyroid's ability to make hormones if you're not getting enough iodine.

Soybeans are one of the crops that are being genetically modified. Since 1997 GMO soybeans are being used in an increasing number of products.

Dr. Kaayla Daniel, author of The Whole Soy Story, points out thousands of studies linking soy to malnutrition, digestive distress, immune-system breakdown, thyroid dysfunction, cognitive decline, reproductive disorders and infertility—even cancer and heart disease. Here is just a sampling of the health effects that have been linked to soy consumption:

Breast cancer

Brain damage

Infant abnormalities

Thyroid disorders

Kidney stones

Immune system impairment

Severe, potentially fatal food allergies

Impaired fertility

Danger during pregnancy and nursing

Final thoughts on Soy: Soy is terrible – contains trypsin inhibitors, is a source of xenoestrogens, even if it's organic, and if it's GMO, it also comes with a lot of glyphosate and other pesticide residues. Avoid it like the black plague.

#4 Empty Calorie Foods

Empty calorie foods are primarily made up of solid fats and/or added sugars. Foods with empty calories can add to your overall caloric intake but offer little to no nutritional value. Empty calories foods such as sweets, sodas and other sweetened beverages are a rich source of sugar. It seems these highly addictive foods taste delicious but can eventually take years off your life and add pounds to your waistline. Eating clean and loaded your body with the needed health fats would benefit your body. Organic meats are always best. Try to eat more organic beef, wild fish, eggs, free-range chicken, good quality protein powders along with avocado, coconut, nuts and seeds, real butter, raw cheese and other organic dairy products.

#5 Sugary Foods

Eating sugar is making your adrenal glands work harder. Stop indirectly making your adrenal gland producing extra cortisol to fight the excess sugar.

There's no way to sugarcoat the truth — Americans are eating more sugar than ever before. Researchers from the University of North Carolina at Chapel Hill determined that, on average, Americans are consuming 83 more calories per day from caloric sweeteners than they did in 1977. And those extra 83 calories a day turn into a whopping 2,490 calories per month.

Sugar addiction is nothing to joke about. Once you're hooked, cravings can be very hard to fight against, leading you down a never ending movement towards obesity and other health problems. Studies are showing that in some people and animals, the brain can react to sugar very much like it can to drugs and alcohol. That's why when you initially cut added sugars from your diet, you might feel deprived for a few days. "When your body is overloaded with waste, you feel more uncomfortable when not eating that food," Fuhrman says. "It's like stopping coffee."

Besides research showing that amazing not-so-innocent sweet tooth could be doing serious damage to your health, leading to weight gain, high blood pressure and cholesterol levels and an increased risk for diabetes. Matter of a fact, Dr. Joel Fuhrman, author of The End of Dieting, says eating too much sugar should be considered just as dangerous as smoking cigarettes. "A diet with sugar and high glycemic index foods promotes all the leading causes of death in America," he says. "I don't see value in cutting out sugar for a few days and then going back to eating it, but I do see value in cutting it out permanently."

#6 Caffeine

Caffeine adds stress to your adrenal glands and the endocrine system. Caffeine will stimulate you adrenals causing them to adrenaline and cortisol in the exact same way as they do during a 'fight or flight' reaction. Caffeine gives you a false boost in energy before the fall to fatigue.

Your thyroid is very sensitive to stimulants. It only confuses your already overworked system.

If you must have coffee, try to limit it to one cup of coffee a day.

As for caffeinated soda, this beverage is a loaded with empty calories, a crazy amount of sugar and then top if off with the caffeine. You can purchase soda water without sodium and squeeze a lemon or lime into it.

#7 Processed Foods

Plain and simple, packaged foods have added preservatives and few nutrients. Chips, cookies, cereals, crackers — foods that come in a bag or box that have been pre-made at a facility.

Cook at home using whole ingredients as nature intended them. I understand this isn't always possible but it's an excellent goal to aim for.

The less you eat packaged foods made of who knows what, the more they begin to taste too salty or become unappetizing in general.

#7 Dairy and Gluten

Most people don't realize that they have a very common food allergies to gluten and dairy. A1 casein is a protein found in cow's milk. The A1 casein and gluten both can cause Leaky Gut Syndrome. This will increase inflammation and tax your already low hormone producing thyroid gland. When you have a "Leaky gut" it allows particles to leak from your digestive tract and travel freely through your bloodstream. This puts your immune system on high alert to neutralize all of these threats. After a while of the constant abuse from your leaky gut and eventually puts your body in a state of chronic inflammation and next setting you on the path to develop an autoimmune disease where your immune system becomes so stressed and confused that it begins attacking your own tissue by mistake. So the next time you go to eat that cheeseburger keep in mind that since you have a leaky gut that was originally caused by gluten and dairy consumption, your willingly allowing their proteins to travel freely into your bloodstream, where they trigger an attack from your immune system. I use ghee for cooking very frequently. The clarifying process also removes casein. I also use coconut milk. In my research, these are a safer way to eat dairy if you must any type of raw dairy – milk, butter, cheese, cream, sour cream, cream cheese, ice cream, heavy cream, yogurt and any type of pasteurized grass-fed dairy of cream, butter, and ghee.

So what's good for my thyroid health?

So, all this gloom and doom about what foods hinder thyroid function — what about those that promote this important butterfly shaped gland?

Let's get this thyroid to function properly and by doing so you will need a mixture of vitamins and minerals, which you can get from the following foods.

8 Foods That Promote Healthy Thyroid Function

Ocean fish and sea vegetables are both an excellent source of iodine. Iodine is key in producing adequate amounts of thyroid hormone. It helps in balancing the metabolism — the process of converting food to energy.

Nuts are loaded with nutrients and protein. Since many of them also contain the antioxidant selenium, I often recommend them for my thyroid patients. Selenium protects your immune system and thyroid, while aiding in the process of converting iodine from food into a usable nutrient. Brazil nuts have the highest concentration of selenium.

Carrots and sweet potatoes are packed with vitamin A, which boosts the immune system. Since many thyroid disorders result in autoimmune disorders such as Hashimoto's or Graves' disease, vitamin A is a must-have.

Organic dairy is an easy way to consume your body's much-needed amount of vitamin D. This vitamin is crucial in maintaining healthy cells that allow for stable thyroid function. Organic dairy also contains optimal amounts of calcium, protein, and iodine.

Beans are chock-full of nutrients that your body craves. In addition to iodine, they are rich in fiber, which helps to stop constipation, a common problem with thyroid malfunction.

Organic beef is loaded with zinc. Like iodine, zinc aids in the process of producing thyroid hormones. Zinc deficiencies can, in turn, prevent the body from making the proper amount of hormones needed for energy.

Bananas contain magnesium, which almost all of my patients need more of. Low levels of magnesium spell trouble for a previously functional thyroid and since so many people are low on this nutrient, upping their daily intake is often an easy fix for regaining energy.

Tomatoes are an excellent source of methylsulfonylmethane (MSM) and vitamins. MSM contains a specific bioavailable sulfur, which is a compound that promotes thyroid function.

Dieting for Your Thyroid

When it comes down to it, the proper diet for our thyroid is one that has balance. We need to constantly be incorporating a healthy amount of the three major sources of macronutrients:

Quality Proteins

Healthy Fats

Healthy Carbohydrates

The mix here is important, and by purchasing my cookbook A survivors cookbook guide to kicking hypothyroidism booty, I will show you exactly how and what you should be working each day into your diet so that you start healing your health. Break that cycle, start eating to cater to your thyroid and replenish your life.

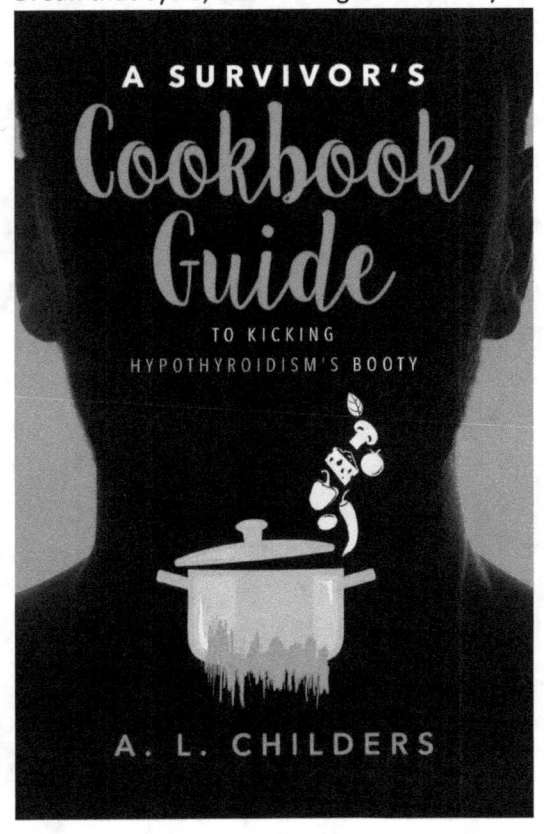

16 Fluorinated Drugs that CRASH Your Thyroid

Top Fluorinated Drugs that crash your thyroid.

Atovastatin, citalopram, dexamethasone, escitalopram, fluconazole, flunisolide, fluoxetine, Fluoroquinolone antibiotics (ciprofloxacin, levofloxacin) , fluticasone, fluvastatin, fluvoxamine, lansoprazole, midazolam, paroxetine, flurazepam

Fluoride displaces iodine in your body and over time that could reduce your thyroid hormone. A very common cause for hypothyroidism, depression, mood disorders and anxiety.

Avoid all sources of fluoride

As I've mentioned in every one of my books and on blog website. Fluoride suppresses the thyroid and can be one of the leading causes of your hypothyroidism. We all are unique. Start drinking filtered water, avoid soft drinks, use fluoride-free toothpaste, use a shower filter, and throw away non-stick cookware. Keep in mind that coffee and tea naturally contain fluoride.

Surely by now you can see the dangers of fluoride consumption. I know, many statements have been made from health officials that fluoride is safe and natural, this isn't the case. Sodium fluoride is being added to many municipal drinking water sources. Fluoride is not safe, and it builds up in our bones and our soft tissue as well as our brains. This will certainly leave us open to major health consequences later.

Fluoride is everywhere. In our toothpastes, tap water, infant formulas, bottle water, prescription drugs, its used to dust crops with, they also use it as a fumigant and put it in pesticides.

Did you know that?

In 1955, Crest became the first fluoride toothpaste.

Fluoride calcifies the penal gland

Fluoride is so toxic that it is considered hazardous waste by the EPA

Hilter fluorinated the water in the concentration camps to sedate the prisoners and lower their IQ's

Fluoride is one of the same ingredients in both rat poison and Prozac.

Fluoride is linked to cancer, lower IQ's, brain damage in babies, cancer in various forms and thyroid problems.

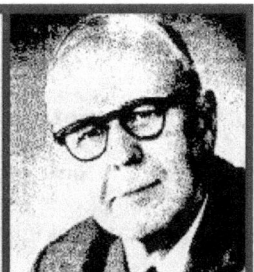

"I know of absolutely no, and I mean absolutely NO means of prevention, that would save so many lives as simply to stop fluoridation. Or, don't start it where it is otherwise going to be started. There, you might save 30,000 or 40,000 lives a year. Cancer lives ... That's an awful lot of lives a year."

Dr. Dean Burk, Ph.D
(34 Years - The National Cancer Institute)
Judicial Hearing, January 14, 1982

Homemade Tooth Powder Recipe

Ingredients

4 tablespoons Bentonite clay

2 teaspoons baking soda

1 ½ teaspoons finely ground unrefined sea salt

½ teaspoons clove powder

1 teaspoon ground Ceylon cinnamon

5-10 drops of peppermint essential oil

¾ teaspoons activated charcoal –

Directions

Using a stainless steel or plastic spoon, mix all ingredients in a clean glass jar. To use, add a little to a wet toothbrush and brush as normal.

Natural Peppermint Toothpaste

1/2 cup coconut oil

3 Tablespoons of baking soda

15 drops of peppermint food grade essential oil

Melt to soften the coconut oil. Mix in other ingredients and stir well. Place your mixture into small glass jar. Allow it to cool completely. When ready to use just dip toothbrush in and scrape small amount onto bristles.

Chapter 4

Is your Hypothyroidism Self Sabotaging your Workouts?

We all know that regular exercise is an important part of your overall health. Exercise burns calories to prevent weight gain and helps speed up your metabolism. It is also a releases endorphins to give you those mood-enhancing chemicals. What if I told you that exercise can cause adrenal crashes due to your already high cortisol issues? You could be stressing your thyroid out even more and not even realizing it. Are you exercising but not getting any results? Are you still gaining weight, feeling constantly fatigued, irritable and moody and often battling some other sort of sickness? You could be actually stressing your body more out by over-exercising.

The magic word here is cortisol.

Cortisol, a steroid hormone produced by the adrenal gland. It is released in response to stress. When you are stressed, your body releases certain "fight-or-flight" stress hormones that are produced in the adrenal glands: cortisol, norepinephrine and epinephrine. Staying stressed raises your cortisol levels and your body actually resists weight loss. Your body thinks times are hard and you might starve, so it hoards the fat you eat or what you have presently on your body. Cortisol will grab fat from your butt and hips, and move it to your abdomen which has more cortisol receptors. Hello there Mrs. Muffin Top!

Today most of us are in a chronic stress state. However, our body don't know the difference between car troubles, relationship issues, debt, work pressure and truly life-threatening stress. This is why our body still ready to defend and reacts exactly the same as it always has done.

Over-exercising can:

Deplete hormones necessary for the functioning of the body

Cause gradual bone loss

Increase injuries

Cause cramping of muscles

Add to inflammation

Increase healing time

Affect cardiac function

Affect blood flow

Decrease the ability of muscles to use fatty acids as a source of energy

Reduce endurance

Here are a few things you can start to incorporate into your life:

1. Limit your caffeine to 200 milligrams a day. (This is equal to about one 12 oz. cup of coffee) In this book, I do list alternative things you can drink that doesn't have caffeine but if you must drink coffee or have caffeine try to limit it to 12oz.'s

2. Start eating a true AIP Keto diet. In doing this you will avoid simple carbs, processed foods, and refined grains, and get plenty of high-quality protein, healthy fats and great vegetables. Look for my book, ***Beyond the Dish: Fix your gut, strengthen your immunity and fight inflammation with this autoimmune approach to Keto.*** Make sure you get with your health care provider before changing your diet in anyway. For example: People with kidney problems and there are people who have protein intolerances. Always, always check with your health care provider 1st.

3. Its okay to say NO! Take time to relax, take a nap, distress and recuperate.

4. Start building your endurance back slowly.

5. Get a heart rate monitor and use it. Know your heart rate comfort zone.

6. Listen to your body. How do you feel the next day? Do you need an extra day to recover?

7. Set realistic goals, one step at a time and don't get discouraged.

8.   Try a Low-impact aerobics workout. Something to get your heart rate up and your lungs going without putting too much pressure on your joints, which is important because joint pain is another common hypothyroidism symptom.

9. Strength training is good. Strength training builds muscle mass, and muscle burns more calories than fat, even when you're at rest.

10. Get some sleep!

Just think how great it's going to feel when you are as healthy on the inside as you look on the outside! The ultimate goal isn't to look fit but to be fit.

How can I lose weight seems to be the most frequently asked question that I hear?

It seemed no matter what diet I tried, I couldn't lose the weight. No matter what exercise I tried, I couldn't shed the weight. What I was missing and what I didn't figure out until much later is that there were many things at play with my weight loss battle. The thyroid medication that I was taking was synthetic T4. I needed my T3 to be converted as well. See, my T3 was my energy hormone and I suffered from this horrible imbalance of my T4 not converting to T3 which lead to my adrenal fatigue. My system was so over worked, I had a lack of nutrients and my body was severely imbalanced. The adrenal fatigue put my body in a battle and my cortisol levels were out of this world! Cortisol add fat around my mid-section. So, the harder I exercised, the more "cortisol"-fat added to my stomach. Then let's mention the leaky gut. My gut played a vital role in my autoimmunity. 95% of all thyroid diseases are autoimmune. Most often undiagnosed. I needed to get my gut fixed. The only way I was going to start to put my Hashimoto's in remission is to start working on my gut. The 70% of my immune system is manufactured in my gut. Like an onion, I started to work on each layer that needed to be addressed, peeling it back, layer by layer. Did I have food sensitives? Many people have food sensitives continue to eat these foods that causes a leaky gut, candida and ph imbalances. Gluten, dairy, soy, eggs and processed foods are just to name a few. Also, no matter how much I worked on my foods and exercise. It wasn't going do me any good if I continued to use household cleaners, aluminum under arm deodorants and fluoride toothpastes. The list can go on and one. I needed to start reading labels and not allow these toxins on my body. I was fighting an uphill battle for my life. I started by the elimination process. Uncovered what foods bothered me, fixed my gut, slowed down my exercise and switched my medication many times. I started eating clean, fermented veggies, low carb and healthy high fat. Reading food labels, if it was artificial or made in a lab I avoided it. If I couldn't eat it, I didn't put it on my body. I avoided all environmental toxins like the plague. I added vital vitamins and minerals that my body was missing and probiotics. This wasn't a "diet" it was a lifestyle change. A complete overhaul of my life in every aspect. I had to start listening to my body, and not one of those a dietary theories. I couldn't force foods that didn't agree with me on myself because someone else thought they were healthy. Dietary theories are meant to be a starting point, your body will give you further directions. This is what led me to writing my books on Hypothyroidism. Recipes that I've used and created for your Mind, body and spirit. These recipes not only nourish your body but feed your spirit. This was my secret to my success to my weight loss.

What will yours be?

I added more things like:

Olives

Avocado

Cooked Cruciferous vegetables (Limit this to no more than 2x per week)

Fermented foods

Fatty fish (e.g., wild-caught salmon trout, tuna and mackerel.)

Chicken and Turkey (organic hormone & Antibiotic free)

Grass Fed Beef

Leafy greens

Nitrate free bacon

Nuts, such as walnuts and almonds

Seeds, such as pumpkin, chia and flax

Coconut Flour, Almond Flour and hemp seeds

Chia Seeds

Kelp and seaweed

Celtic or Himalayan sea salt

Coconut

Coconut oil

Organic butter (preferably Grass fed)

Ghee

Bone Broth

Eggs: Look for pastured or omega-3 whole eggs. (if you don't have a food allergy)

Cheese: Unprocessed cheese (cheddar, goat, cream, blue or mozzarella).

Fish oil (EPA/DHA)

Magnesium

Vitamin B Complex

Vitamin C

Vitamin D3

Zinc

Ancient Nutrition- Bone Broth Collagen Loaded with Bone Broth Co-Factors

Take your medication in the morning with 16oz of warm freshly squeezed lemon water

2. If you drink coffee, drink it in the morning. Wait 1 hour after your medication and please let it be bullet proof coffee! I make bullet proof green tea. Same concept as bullet proof coffee but without the caffeine. I do have a section in this book why your morning coffee is bad for you.

3. Drink a glass of water before every meal

4. Don't drink your calories. Don't waste your calories. Most of everything is a calorie. Read labels.

5. Eat a protein at every meal (Remember: Soy & fake foods are not healthy proteins!!)

6. Avoid gluten

7. Avoid bad carbs.

Refined grains like white bread, white rice and enriched pasta

Processed foods such as cake, candy, cookies and chips

White potatoes

Sweetened soft drinks

Sugar

8. READ food labels (stay away from fake, made in a lab, made by man, processed or artificial foods aka Frankenstein foods meaning they are not real) Remember if it can sit on the shelf for a long time, it certainly can sit in your body the same way.

9. Size does matter. Learn your portion sizes

10. Get your good fats in!

Avocados

Walnuts

Almonds

Nut and seed butters. ...

Olives

Olive oil

Ground flaxseed

Salmon

11. No fried foods, no fast food

12. Eat a real breakfast!

No Bake Dairy Free Sugar Free Overnight Oats

Ingredients

3 cups Bob's Red Mill Gluten-Free Old Fashioned Rolled Oats

3 cups unsweetened almond milk

3 tablespoon of chia seeds

1/2 teaspoon of vanilla extract

Instructions

In a large bowl stir together all ingredients except fruit toppings.

Let stand for 30 minutes.

Divide mixture into 4 mason jars, about 3/4 cup each or 6 mason jars, about 1/2 cup each.

Add fruit toppings to each if desired.

Cover and refrigerate overnight.

Quinoa Breakfast bowl

1 cup of cooked quinoa

1/2 cup of unsweetened almond milk

1/2 teaspoon of cinnamon

1/3 cup of blueberries

Cook quinoa according to directions

Add almond milk to warm quinoa

Mix in cinnamon & blue berries

Have you ever wondered why people respond differently to diets?

In the last fifty years what has changed in our society? We have the same predisposition genetics as our grandparents. We are unique and come in all different shapes and sizes.

We can't blame is all on genetics being unhealthy solely on the DNA that was passed down to us. Everyone's genetic makeup is different. It's like your fingerprints.

I was always the tall, skinny, freckled faced, flat chested, flat butt girl in school. I remember being plagued at school for being too skinny. Having no shape. While other school mates were well endowed with large boobs, hippy hips and a nice rounder booty. Our metabolisms certainly dictate how we use energy and our genetics can dictate how we are shaped but what has started to interests me more-so lately is why we store fat on certain areas of our bodies when others don't.

These questions have confused and frustrated people and health care practitioners for decades. But why is it so confusing? One thing we have learned is each of us are unique and have our very own biochemistry that sets us apart from everyone else. Although we might share the same common traits and perhaps the same overlapping metabolic tendencies. We can't continue to say that one-size-fits-all when it comes to our very own unique body chemistry. There are over 7 billion people on this planet and we come in all different shapes, colors and sizes. With this being said wouldn't you think the one-size-fits-all- approach to losing weight wouldn't work since we are we are all unique.

Why it is that one person can eat all they want and never gain an inch, while someone else gains weight just looking at food? The fact is some people are wired to simply burn fat better than others. There are sneaky little things in your body that can halt your weight loss success.

Where you store your body fat isn't a topic most of us women like to discuss but I feel it is one that will enlighten you and help you more on your journey to a better healthier you.

Every cell in our body responds to the foods we eat, the products we put on our bodies and the household chemicals that we come in contact with every day. Although some of us were born with the predisposition genetics as our parents that gives us our hair color, eye color, height and if we are pear shaped, apple shaped, straight or hourglass this doesn't mean we can't win the battle when it comes to our hormones. Our hormones have a direct impact on every major system in our body. Remember our bodies love balance. Everything has a domino effect so we have to try to figure-out that balance in what our individual body needs are. Whether it be the more fiber , fixing our gut, helping our skin get more moisture, speeding up our metabolism so we can get out of that fat storage mode and into the fat burning mode.

After researching many hours on this topic, I've found that where your body stores fat is hint to what is going on with you internally with your hormones. As our hormone levels change with age, pregnancy, exercise, eating habits, or other life events, fat adjusts itself to our every changing hormonal events and places itself in different area's in our body. Our hormones have a direct impact on how much body fat we store and where it is stored on our bodies. Wouldn't it be wonderful to know what approach to take to fix those thunder thighs or that muffin top?   Now even with this information it's just a stepping stone of knowledge to better equip you a healthier you. So what exactly does it mean to have fat stored in certain areas of your body and not others?

Love handles/belly: Love handles often means that you are way too stressed out and when you're stressed out it raises your cortisol levels. It could also be an indicator that you might have adrenal fatigue. Cortisol adds fat around my mid-section. You are eating too much sugar where you become insulin resistant. If your body is in constant elevated levels of insulin (a hormone that regulates the metabolism of carbohydrates in the bloodstream) it will accumulate around your mid-section. A lack of sleep also may lead to metabolic issues and help encourage those love handles. It also could mean you have elevated estrogen levels and more insulin production. So what do you need to do? Stop eating crap, those processed carbs and avoid sugar, even the fake sugars which are even more horrible for you. You should also go easy on the exercise, sometimes if you exercise more it adds more cortisol to your body so you are fighting a losing battle, try yoga, more sleep, meditation, Pilates, planks, lifting weights and walking are good ways to start. Don't forget fat gained around the waist is dangerous in terms of it increases the risk of heart disease, diabetes and other chronic diseases. **My book reset your Thyroid. This is a 21-day Meal plan to reset your thyroid and jump start your weight loss journey.** It is filled with 21 breakfast recipes, 21 lunch recipes and 21 dinner recipes. They are packed full of nutrients, healthy fats and proteins. All are easy to make and I've done all the thinking for you! Or you can start eating a true **AIP Keto diet**. In doing this you will avoid simple carbs, processed foods, and refined grains, and get plenty of high-quality protein, healthy fats and great vegetables. Look for my book, **Beyond the Dish: Fix your gut, strengthen your immunity and fight inflammation with this autoimmune approach to Keto.** Make sure you get with your health care provider before changing your diet in anyway. For example: People with kidney problems and there are people who have protein intolerances. Always, always check with your health care provider 1st.

Thighs: Sometimes it's our genetic bone structure that was passed down from our parents that gives us more hips or fatter thighs than the next person and other times it can mean that we have elevated estrogen levels. This is the female sex hormone. Thigh fat is a little harder to burn off than belly fat. You can also have fluid retention in your thighs. So many think that fluid retention only takes place only in the abdomen but that isn't true It actually occurs all over your body. So what do you need to do? Start drinking your daily needed allowance of water. Your body weight and divide it by two. That's the least amount of water to drink per day and please don't drink it all in one sitting. There is a think called water toxicity and it will kill you. Space out your water consumption. Choose better skin care products in my blog 21 Successful Tips on Clean Beauty Swaps. I share with your skin care products are healthier. You want to avoid chemicals such as BPA (that can be found in plastic containers, water bottles and pretty much anything plastic unless it states BPA FREE) , parabens or phthalates. Your food should be 100% organic and you most defiantly should be avoiding all soy products like the black plague. Let's not forget that getting in a good night's sleep will also help to improve your estrogen levels. In my book, A Survivor's Cookbook Guide to Kicking Hypothyroidism's Booty, I've included clean food recipes, recipes for your home and body that are super easy to make, who doesn't want a healthier home?

Back of Arms: This could mean that you have lower testosterone levels as well as an excess insulin. Women do have a small amount of testosterone in our adrenal glands and ovaries although this is thought as a male hormone. Start eating more avocados, as in healthy fats and fatty fish such as salmon can help improve this area. Try to avoid all red meat and all dairy products. Start trying to lift some weights. Building muscle through weight lifting can and may also increase testosterone levels.

Upper Back: This could mean you have lower levels of Thyroxine and higher levels of insulin. Thyroxine is a thyroid hormone that plays a role with your metabolism and calorie burning rate and this hormone is secreted into our bloodstream. You can help boost your thyroxine naturally by eating foods such as shellfish, seafood and cruciferous vegetables, avoiding gluten and soy, and increasing healthy fat intake.

Our metabolism does not decide to burn or store body fat based on calories. It makes these decisions based on the hormones those calories trigger. That is why the quality of calories matters so much….higher-quality calories trigger body-fat-burning hormones while low-quality calories trigger body-fat-storing hormones.

– The Smarter Science of Slim

As the conclusion, Body fat is important necessity for life. It is our source of energy and it stores some much needed nutrients, a major ingredient in brain tissue. Moreover, it provides a padding to protect internal organs and insulates the body against the cold. But yet, getting too fat (more than 30 percent body fat in females and 25 percent in males) can be dangerous and is associated with increased risk of disease and premature death, regardless of where the fat is stored in the body. As an American society, we are tipping the scales to the point that obesity is now a national health epidemic.

Think about this each time you eat, hormones are released into your body and the type of calories consumed (i.e. fat, carbohydrates or protein) determines which hormones are released and where it is placed throughout your body. The only way to achieve your goal is to start eating to cater to your body's needs. Along with proper exercise. I've given you all solutions to fight that fat storage on those certain areas of your body part. I suggest eating a particular way to combat the hormone imbalances and I know for a fact that if you put forth the effort it will be easily attainable.

Metabolic Syndrome

There are many studies showing that a lower -carb diet does improve most cases metabolic syndrome such as blood lipids, insulin levels, HDL-cholesterol, LDL particle size and fasted blood sugar levels

When I first began a Keto lifestyle change, my body fully adapted and started using fat as the primary source of my energy.

If you have   any pre-existing kidney or diabetic conditions– as the higher intake of proteins will put strain on your kidneys. Always check with your health care provider before starting any new eating plan.

I found out that my bad cholesterol went down and it increased my good cholesterol went up.

I started to get my mindset right and decided on a more realistic, healthy approach at losing my body fat.

Water Boosts Metabolism

Lots of people don't realize the importance of drinking enough water every day and how it can impact both your health and your weight loss efforts. Water is involved in every type of cellular process in your body, and when you're dehydrated, they all run less efficiently — and that includes your metabolism.

"Your metabolism is basically a series of chemical reactions that take place in your body. Staying hydrated keeps those chemical reactions moving smoothly. Being slightly dehydrated can have an impact on your metabolism.

Aim for at least 100 ounces a day – especially in the first couple of weeks until your body adjusts.

(Necessary internet disclaimer: there is such a thing as too much water so don't get silly about it)

To make it a little easier to calculate how much water to drink every day, here are the recommended amounts for a range of weights. Remember to adjust for your activity level.

Weight	Ounces of Water Daily
100 pounds	67 ounces
110 pounds	74 ounces
120 pounds	80 ounces
130 pounds	87 ounces
140 pounds	94 ounces
150 pounds	100 ounces
160 pounds	107 ounces
170 pounds	114 ounces
180 pounds	121 ounces
190 pounds	127 ounces
200 pounds	134 ounces
210 pounds	141 ounces
220 pounds	148 ounces
230 pounds	154 ounces
240 pounds	161 ounces
250 pounds	168 ounces

Life is an experiment. Be kind to yourself. People really don't know what you are going through. Be patient, love yourself and step forward without judgement on those who have no clue. Reach for happiest with every breath you take. Trust your heart. Keep your faith and walk ahead!—A.L. Childers

In case you get hungry between meals, here are some healthy, approved snacks:

Fatty meat or fish.

Cheese.

A handful of nuts or seeds.

Cheese with olives.

1–2 hard-boiled eggs.

90% dark chocolate.

A low-carb milk shake with almond milk, cocoa powder and nut butter.

Celery with salsa and guacamole.

Discover-The Truth Behind Why You Can't Shed Those Hypothyroidism Pounds!

It certainly can be frustrating after a few weeks of hard work, you step on the scale only to find the number hasn't budged at all. Things you might not realize your doing can counteract your hard working efforts to shed those unsightly pounds. More often than none you can't figure out why you moved that muffin top. Let's be realistic you won't start to look like that celebrity or fitness model unless you can clone them. Everyone's genetic makeup is different. It's like your finger prints. NO two sets are the same. Even identical twins are one egg that split but they are very different in more ways than one. The fact is some people are wired to simply burn fat better than others. Don't raise that white flag and give in, just yet. See there are a few sneaky little things that can secretly halt your weight loss success without you even realizing. I'm going to try to help you get to the root of your problem. I want you to make changes in your life that are doable and successful.

First of all, dieting can be stressful. Never restrict your calories that will produce stress hormones and your fat cells will increase the amount of abdominal fat because your body is thinking your starving. Next, keep a food diary. I want you to write down everything you stick in your mouth, everything you drink, how many ounces and even look at the body products you use, house hold chemicals and the exercise that you do. Do this for a week. Now, you will have an overall picture of what you are doing and how you need to adjust and change things.

So let's get down to the nitty-gritty of it all.

Looking at the big picture. Like an onion, you must start to work on each layer and see what needs to be addressed, peeling it back, layer by layer.

You have the power to make a difference in your life. You've always had the power. No one can force you to become more aware of what you put on your body and what you put in your body. What you eat is just as important as what you put on your body. Adjusting your life, reading labels and catering to your specific health needs isn't easy but it will benefit you in the long run. This is one of the smartest decisions that you can make. Not only will you start to look and feel better but think of the medical cost that you could be saving your future self.

Most importantly before you begin to read this ... Embrace your body. Whatever size and shape you are always think positive about yourself.

Do you have an underlying health condition that will make you gain weight?

There are other health conditions other than hypothyroidism that will contribute to weight gain. Whatever other medical issues you might have don't feel you are a lost case because you can take this in consideration. What you need to do is research about your medical condition on how to lose weight or get with a registered dietitian who can help you create a meal plan just for your specific body needs.

17 Underlying health conditions/reasons that add can weight

Underactive thyroid, Diabetes treatment, Ageing, Steroid treatments, Cushing's syndrome, Stress, chronic fatigue syndrome, Fluid retention, fibromyalgia, Polycystic ovary syndrome (PCOS), Menopause, Depression, heart disease, hormonal disorders, sleep disorders, Adrenal fatigue, Cellular toxicity, leaky gut, Candida, No motivation , No extra time

Are you on a medication that makes you gain weight?

Certain medications, notably steroids, and also some antidepressants, antipsychotics, high blood pressure drugs, allergy medication, birth control, and seizure medications has been linked to adding the extra lbs. to your waistline. Keep in mind we are all different not everybody will experience the same side effects if any with medications.

Don't ever stop taking any medications without first consulting your doctor. You're on that medication for a reason and it just may be critical to your health. Please always consult with your doctor so they can try to help you figure out what's going on but be honest. Don't go into the doctor's office saying your gaining weight and you can't figure it out knowing you had that diet coke & Twinkie for breakfast!

Here is your check list!

1. Are you eating to cater to your body's needs? For example: if you hypothyroidism, are you eating to cater to that? In this book, I have given you the blueprint to eat to cater to your thyroid.

2. Are you on medications that make you gain weight? If you don't know, research the medications and then consult with your doctor to see what can be done to help you shed those lbs. Maybe change your medications?

3. Do you have an underlying health condition that has a history of weight gain in patients? If so, research on how other people have successfully lost weight with that medical condition, join a support group if need be to get ideas and tips and extra support.

4. Have you taken antibiotics? Did you know that it has been proven by scientist that it can take up to a year to fix your gut flora after taken antibiotics?

5. Did you know artificial sweeteners will stale or mess up your gut flora, causing an inflammatory response and your body will become resistant to weight loss? Read labels. Avoid all those fake sugars. No diet drinks, processed food or artificial anything! If it's made in a lab, avoid it.

6. Are you drinking plenty of water? Not drinking enough water or being dehydrated will halt your weight loss. Take your weight divide by two and that is how many ounces you should be drinking each day. Here is a simple yet effective flavored water drink of mine.

Water Boosts Metabolism

I've already covered this but let me go over it again. Lots of people don't realize the true importance of drinking enough water every day and how it can impact both your health and your weight loss efforts. "Water's involved in every type of cellular process in your body, and when you're dehydrated, everything runs less efficiently. It slows down your metabolism.

Your metabolism is basically a series of chemical reactions that take place in your body. Staying hydrated keeps those chemical reactions moving smoothly. If you are even slightly dehydrated that will affect your metabolism.

Aim for at least 100 ounces a day – especially in the first couple of weeks until your body adjusts.

7. Eat breakfast- breakfast is the most important meal to the day. Never ever skip breakfast. The right breakfast foods can help you concentrate, give you energy and get your metabolism moving.   In my book : A survivors cookbook guide to kicking hypothyroidism booty I have over 25 amazing breakfast recipes that will teach how to make the perfect overnight oats to make your mornings totally effortless, quick and you'll have no reason to not eat breakfast again!

No Bake Dairy Free Sugar Free Overnight Oats

Ingredients

3 cups Bob's Red Mill Gluten-Free Old Fashioned Rolled Oats

3 cups unsweetened almond milk

3 tablespoon of chia seeds

1/2 teaspoon of vanilla extract

Instructions

In a large bowl stir together all ingredients except fruit toppings.

Let stand for 30 minutes.

Divide mixture into 4 mason jars, about 3/4 cup each or 6 mason jars, about 1/2 cup each.

Add fruit toppings to each if desired.

Cover and refrigerate overnight.

8. Replace a meal with a smoothie or a fresh juice!

Healing Juice Recipe

Ingredients

1 small head romaine

1 organic green apple

3 stalks organic celery

½ organic cucumber

1 lemon

1/2 fresh ginger or turmeric

Directions:

Cut everything to fit into your juicer. Drink and enjoy. Viola!

Audrey's Thyroid Juice Elixir

1/3 bunch dandelion greens

2/3 cup parsley

3 celery stalks

2 inches fresh ginger or turmeric

1 apple

1 lemon

1/2 cup of fresh flesh from a coconut

Add 1 cup of fresh coconut juice

Directions:

Cut everything to fit into your juicer. Drink and enjoy. Viola!

Be creative with your smoothies. If they are too thick, add more liquid, if they are too thin for your liking add less liquid. Play with the ingredients. Make a smoothie that you know you're going to drink. Every single smoothie has celery in it. The reason why celery is in every smoothie is it has super health benefits that range from reducing inflammation, regulates the body's alkaline balance, aids digestion, reduces "bad" cholesterol, reduces bloating, helps to prevent ulcers, lowers blood pressure, amps up your sex life, cancer fighter, excellent source of antioxidants and beneficial enzymes, in addition to vitamins and minerals such as vitamin K, vitamin C, potassium, folate and vitamin B6.

I also suggest that you go with an all-natural vegan, gluten free, dairy free, lactose free, no fillers, no synthetic nutrients, no artificial flavors or sweeteners, no preservatives , no pea protein and soy free protein mix. This is why I use Raw Meal, Garden of life brand products. No they are not endorsing me to say this. I picked this brand after a long research. I am sure there are other brands just as good as this brand but I prefer this brand.

Become mindful and read labels. You want to stay clear of hidden poisons that can be in your protein powders. Here are 3 to be on the lookout for to avoid.

Soy Protein Isolate

Soy protein has been a main ingredient in many protein powders for a while. Soy has been found to be toxic to the digestive system and creates the following concerns:

Disrupts thyroid and endocrine function

Interferes with leptin sensitivity which can cause metabolic syndrome

Throws off estrogen and testosterone balance

Blocks the body's ability to access key minerals like iron, zinc, calcium, and magnesium

It is also estimated that soy is over 95% genetically modified, and one of the most pesticide ridden crops on the market.

This makes any non-organic soy protein (especially isolate) found in protein powders, indigestible and toxic to the human physiology.

Whey Protein Isolate

Whey protein can be a quality protein. Not many on the market are good to digest. If whey came from conventionally raised cows that have been fed non-organic grains and genetically modified foods, and been injected with antibiotics and hormones, which makes it not a good quality source of protein. You also need to keep in mind that this form of whey in an isolate format is not properly absorbed by the body.

If you do choose a whey protein, it is important to see where the whey has come from. Make sure it is from grass fed cows. Which are nutritionally superior compared to grain fed, and they contain an impressive amino acid and immune-supportive nutrient profile.

Rice Protein

Same as the source of the whey protein, the kicker is where it comes from. Even though rice protein can be an acceptable source of protein but many that are not.

Thanks to a report unveiled earlier in 2014 by Mike Adams, we have been able to discover that there are many rice protein powders on the market that have been heavily contaminated with tungsten, cadmium, and lead. The reason for this high level of contamination is due to sourcing rice from China, where air pollution can trump the "organic" label placed on many products, including rice.

Super Charge Green Smoothie

½ organic cucumber, chopped

2 celery stalks

¼ cup parsley

½ lemon, peeled

½ avocado, peeled and pitted

2 cups of organic romaine lettuce

1 scoop of raw meal- garden of Life

1 cup of coconut water

1 cup of ice

Add all ingredients to blender and blend until smooth. Enjoy!

Blueberry Chocolate Delight

½ cup of frozen blueberries

1 cup of romaine lettuce

2 celery stalks

½ teaspoon of Ceylon Cinnamon

1 scoop of raw meal –garden of life- chocolate flavor

2 tablespoons of almond butter

1 cup of unsweetened nut milk

Add all ingredients to blender and blend until smooth. Enjoy!

Happy Colon Smoothie

1 cup pumpkin puree

2 stalks of celery

1 tablespoon raw honey

½ of a peeled grapefruit

1 cup unsweetened almond milk

2 tablespoon flaxseed meal

½ inch fresh raw ginger

½ teaspoon cinnamon, nutmeg & turmeric

This a delicious, easy drink to make. Add all ingredients into the blender and voila!

9. Do you have chronic candida?

I have a recipe in this book for a parasite and candida drink. One you start healing your gut, adding fermented vegetables, taking a quality probiotic and eating better this will help rid your body of the candida. After you start boosting your immune system and eliminate sugar, alcohol and refined carbohydrates your body will start to heal itself. Remember yeast loves sugar.

10. Do you have parasites?

When we have any of the GI infections listed above (parasite, bacteria, fungal), damage has been (and is being) done to our gut lining. This means that we aren't able to digest and absorb the nutrients from our food, and this negatively affects our tissues and organs. This is why we may likely experience symptoms in other body systems that do not appear to be directly related to the gut.

In terms of weight gain or inability to lose weight, we must remember the cortisol connection. When we have a chronic GI infection, this triggers inflammation and therefore sends the message to our body that we need more cortisol, a primary anti-inflammatory hormone. Cortisol is also a sort of fat storage hormone, so when we are over-producing it, our body holds onto weight (particularly around the mid-section).

11. The Chemical romance that we call food.

Did you know that products we use every day may contain toxic chemicals and has been linked to women's health issues? They are hidden endocrine disruptors and are very tricky chemicals that play havoc on our bodies. "We are all routinely exposed to endocrine disruptors, and this has the potential to significantly harm the health of our youth," said Renee Sharp, EWG's director of research. "It's important to do what we can to avoid them, but at the same time we can't shop our way out of the problem. We need to have a real chemical policy reform." The longer the length of ingredients on your food label means how much more unhealthy it is for you to consume. When an item contains a host of ingredients that most likely you can't even pronounce or remember to spell you can bet your lucky dollar that the natural nutrients are long gone. These highly processed frank n foods are very difficult for the body to break down and some of the chemicals will become stored in your body.

12. Did you know that it takes 26 seconds for the chemicals in personal body care products to enter into your bloodstream? Endocrine disruptors are tricky chemicals that play on our bodies. They increase production of certain hormones; decreasing production of others; imitating hormones; turning one hormone into another; interfering with hormone signaling; telling cells to die prematurely; competing with essential nutrients; binding to essential hormones; accumulating in organs that produce hormones. You can start avoiding these chemicals by starting with detoxifying your beauty routine. If you want to protect your body from the harmful ingredients that are used in most commercial brands, you should check out organic skin care products and organic make-up. Start reading labels and asking questions. Please look for my book **Awareness has Magic.** It is full of DIY recipes for your home, body and spirit.

13. **Do you food allergies?** Many people have food sensitives continue to eat these foods that causes a leaky gut, candida and ph imbalances. Gluten, dairy, soy, eggs and processed foods are just to name a few.

14. **Do you have adrenal fatigue?** The adrenal fatigue put my body in a battle and my cortisol levels were out of this world! Cortisol add fat around my mid-section. So, the harder I exercised, the more "cortisol"-fat added to my stomach.

15. **Do you have a leaky gut?** Then let's mention the leaky gut. My gut played a vital role in my autoimmunity. Most often undiagnosed.

16. **Do you have metabolic syndrome?**

17. Replace Canola oil or other vegetable oils with coconut oil and grass fed butter because those other oils will slow down your weight loss and they will start

to store unwanted body fat. Those genetically modified hydrogenated oils will cause inflammation in your body, along with cellular toxicity.

18. NO SOY products or NO GLUTEN products. Read labels!!!

19. Take THYROID-Boosting vitamins!

Theses Thyroid ESSENTIAL NUTRIENTS: Provides an excellent source of any of these thyroid-boosting nutrients:

Selenium

Zinc

Copper

Iron

20. FREE your home and body of HORMONES, PESTICIDES & TOXINS: These things are thyroid endocrine-disrupting toxins that are found in our conventional food supply along with body products and household chemicals. This means NO BPA, PCBs, dioxins, rBST, PFCs, pesticides, antibiotics, artificial sweeteners, heavy metals, PFOA, chlorine, fluoride, harmful additives or preservatives.

21. No farm raised fish!

Farmed salmon contain 10 times more carcinogenic toxins (PCBs, dioxin, etc.) than wild salmon, according to a study published in the journal Science.

Eating more than one meal of farmed salmon per month contains enough PCBs to raise cancer risk.

Farmed fish are administered more antibiotics by weight than any other livestock.

Seven out of 10 pieces of farmed fish tested had concentrations of cancer-causing PCBs high enough to trigger health warnings from the U.S. Environmental Protection Agency.

22. Stop weighing yourself everyday

Weight loss is a process. If you continue to jump on that scale every day, you will notice higher weight days and lower weight days. If you're exercising and gaining muscle you still could be losing fat and the scales are just not showing it. Go with how your clothes feels. Try taking pictures where you can look at the process.

23. Stop eating all those carbs!

People have food allergies and just don't know it but others are more sensitive to carbs.

Keep a food journal. Write down what you eat, how many carbs and calories you're consuming. You may need to start under 50 grams of carbs per day and try to temporary eliminate fruits. After you go under 50 grams per day if that's not working for you then try 20 grams but let that only be temporary. Just to see if it works. Make sure you're eating healthy organic proteins, healthy fats and leafy green vegetables. Avoid raw cruciferous veggies

 Such as cabbage, kale, Brussels sprouts, broccoli and cauliflower contain natural chemicals called goitrogens (goiter producers) that can interfere with thyroid hormone synthesis.

24. Are you stressed out?

It's sad that sometimes it isn't always enough to just eat healthy and exercise. We need to make sure that our bodies are functioning optimally and that our hormonal environment is favorable. Being stressed all the time keeps the body in a constant state of "fight or flight" – with elevated levels of stress hormones like cortisol. This cortisol is stored around your midsection too. This elevated cortisol levels will increase your hunger and cravings for unhealthy foods. All this chronic stress will have a negative effect on your hormonal environment and in return make you hungrier and halt your weight loss goals.

25. Stop eating crap!

You must throw away all that processed crap and start eating real, nutritious foods. You need to be eating healthy fats, organic proteins and low carb veggies. We want to get your body into an optimal hormonal environment to fat burning mode.

26. Are you getting enough sleep?

Sleep is so important to our heart health and our waist lines. Studies have shown that a lack of sleep correlates with weight gain and obesity. Not getting enough sleep can make us feel hungrier too. Along with feeling tired and less motivated to exercise. Sleep is one of the pillars of health.

27. That diet drink is NOT your friend.

Artificial sweetener are so bad for us and it makes us fat! It can also make us hungry. Avoid any artificial sweetener at all costs.

28. You need to move it or lose it

The right kinds of exercise will improve your bodies hormonal state, increase your muscle mass and boost your serotonin levels with make you feel good. Exercise is important for both your physical and mental health

29. Keep a food journal.

You really need to keep a food journal of everything you stick in your mouth, on your body and chemicals you come in contact with. Write down how many carbs & calories your consuming too. You could be eating too many calories. Losing 1-2 pounds per week is a realistic approach. It takes some longer than others to lose the extra weight and we all can't look like fitness models.

Other idea's to help you in your journey:

Set Up Your Food Storage, Meal prep, Take out all the bad food in your house, go swimming, work your muscles, join a support group, get some sun, get sleep, reduce stress, Eat soluble fibers, Eat mostly whole, unprocessed foods & Drink water a half hour before meals.

This has been my secret to my success to my weight loss.

What will yours be?

I added more things like:

Olives

Avocado

Cooked Cruciferous vegetables (Limit this to no more than 2x per week)

Fermented foods

Fatty fish (e.g., wild-caught salmon trout, tuna and mackerel.)

Chicken and Turkey (organic hormone & Antibiotic free)

Grass Fed Beef

Leafy greens

Nitrate free bacon

Nuts, such as walnuts and almonds

Seeds, such as pumpkin, chia and flax

Coconut Flour, Almond Flour and hemp seeds

Asparagus

Mushrooms.

Zucchini

Cooked cabbage

Any cruciferous vegetables cooked but no more than 2x per week

Cucumber

Lettuce

Tomatoes

Olives

Red, green and orange bell peppers

Onion

Sweet potatoes

Beet root

Chia Seeds

Kelp and seaweed

Celtic or Himalayan sea salt

Coconut

Coconut oil

Organic butter (preferably Grass fed)

Ghee

Bone Broth

Eggs: Look for pastured or omega-3 whole eggs. (If you don't have a food allergy)

Cheese: Unprocessed cheese (cheddar, goat, cream, blue or mozzarella).

Fish oil (EPA/DHA)

Magnesium

Vitamin B Complex

Vitamin C

Vitamin D3

Zinc

Ancient Nutrition- Bone Broth Collagen Loaded with Bone Broth Co-Factors

Studies have shown that this lifestyle change will;

Improve triglyceride levels and cholesterol levels, add in your weight loss, help balance your blood sugar, give your body a better and more reliable energy source, you will feel more energized during the day. Fats are shown to be the most effective molecule to burn as fuel. You will find yourself staying full longer too.

-Day Sample Eating Plan

Breakfast: Overnight Chia Seed Pudding

2 cup coconut milk

1 cup berries

1 scoop grass-fed protein

2 tablespoon chia seeds

1/4 teaspoon cinnamon

Instructions

Add all ingredients except sweetener to a mixing bowl and whisk vigorously to combine. If not blending (which I preferred!), sweeten to taste with maple syrup at this time. If blending, you can sweeten later with maple syrup or dates.

Let rest covered in the fridge overnight or at least 3-5 hours (or until it's achieved a pudding-like consistency).

If blending, add to a blender and blend until completely smooth and creamy, scraping down sides as needed. Sweeten to taste.

Leftovers keep covered in the fridge for 2-3 days, though best when fresh.

Lunch: Greek Salad

1 sliced chicken breast

1 cup organic romaine lettuce

1/4 cup sliced cucumber

1/2 tomato sliced

1 ounce goat cheese

1 tablespoon olive oil

1 tablespoon apple cider vinegar

Grilled salmon with broccoli and cauliflower on white plate Dinner: Organic Meat (bison burger, salmon, chicken)

6 ounces organic meat

1 serving sautéed zucchini

1 serving sautéed sweet potato

Or you can make a casserole dish, something in the crock pot

Stuffed Cabbage Casserole

Ingredients

   1½ lbs. green cabbage

   1⁄3 lb. butter

   1 lb. grass fed ground beef

   1 teaspoon salt

   1 teaspoon onion powder

   ¼ teaspoon ground black pepper

   2 tablespoons tex-mex seasoning

   1 tablespoon white wine vinegar

2/3 lb. shredded cheese, preferably cheddar cheese

1/3 lb. leafy greens or lettuce

Instructions

Preheat oven to 400°F (200°C). Shred the cabbage finely with a sharp knife or in a food processor.

Fry the cabbage in 3 ounces of butter in a large frying pan or a wok on medium-high heat. Fry until soft, but don't let the cabbage turn brown. This can take a little while; roughly 10 minutes.

Add spices and vinegar. Stir and continue to fry for a couple of minutes. Set aside on a plate.

Melt the rest of the butter in the same pan. Sauté the ground beef and fry on medium-high heat until most of the juices have evaporated. Lower the heat to medium-low.

Add cooked cabbage and sauté together with the beef for a minute. Remove from heat and add salt and pepper to taste.

Stir ⅔ of the cheese into the cabbage mix and place in a baking dish.

Sprinkle the rest of the cheese on top and bake for 15–20 minutes or until the cheese browns nicely.

Serve with a green salad.

Cajun Salmon Patties

1 Can Pink salmon, boneless & skinless

2 Tbsp. Coconut Paleo Mayonnaise

1 Large Egg, beaten

2 Tsp Lemon juice

1 Tbsp. Parsley, dried

1/4 Tsp Garlic powder

2 Tbsp. Green onions, chopped

1 tablespoon of Cajun seasoning

1. Drain and flake your salmon in a colander. Transfer the contents to a large mixing bowl, and combine with mayonnaise and an egg to help your recipe bind together.

2. Mix in garlic powder, chopped green onion, and squeeze in 2 teaspoons of lemon juice.

3. Mix in parsley for added flavor and texture.

4. Once all ingredients have been incorporated, it's time to make the patties with your hands. To keep your patties from sticking to your hands, keep a small bowl of water and damp your hands while you form the patties.

5. Once your patties are ready to go, spray a skillet with coconut oil non-stick cooking spray and bring it to medium heat. Place your patties, and cook both sides until they're lightly browned and heated through.

Coconut Paleo Mayonnaise

　2 egg yolks

　1 tsp mustard (this is optional)

　3 tsp lemon juice

　1/2 cup olive oil

　1/2 cup coconut oil

　In a medium bowl (blender, food processor) mix the yolks, mustard, if using, and 1 tsp lemon juice.

　Start whisking vigorously (blender or food processor on low) while dripping the oil very slowly, even drop by drop in the beginning. You're creating an emulsion and if you put too much oil at once, it will separate and will be very hard to save. Whisk non-stop and use a towel under the bowl to help stabilize it.

As you add more oil, the emulsion will form and the mayonnaise will start to thicken and you can pour the oil faster at this point.

When all the oil is incorporated and the mayonnaise is thick, whisk in the rest of the lemon juice and taste your creation. You can season to taste with salt and pepper.

Enjoy without guilt and keep the leftovers in the refrigerator!

Your underlying question needs to be: Why is my body out of balance and how can I help it regain its balance?

Of course your autoimmune disease didn't happen overnight and yes you might have a genetic predisposition towards autoimmunity but science has proven that even if you have a preexisting genetic predisposition towards autoimmunity (meaning it was passed down in your genes from your parents) Our genes are ever changing and are not static . Your genes are wonderful, busy little cells that can be both turned on and turned off by your environmental and lifestyle choices.

Isn't that fantastic? What wonderful news!

You must become your very own investigator. You need to find the root cause of your autoimmunity by uncovering these environmental and lifestyle choices that you've made that has turned on these genes. The small steps that we begin with start to make a difference and I discovered that when you begin to address these five common environmental and lifestyle choices you can start to restore the balance of your immune system and in many change your life completely. Wouldn't it be fantastic if you could begin to reverse your autoimmune disease, improve your quality of life, restore balance to your immune system, off your medications and most importantly become symptom free? This may sound like a distant dream but not one that certainly isn't attainable. You must start to address the root causes of your autoimmune disease. As someone who has battled autoimmune disease myself, it's important to know about that I reversed my autoimmune diseases and you can too.

FACT: The number of people suffering from hypothyroidism continues to rise each year. Levothyroxine is the 4th highest selling drug in the U.S.

FACT: Every Cell in your body responds to your thyroid hormones. These hormones have a direct impact on every major system in your body.

Superfoods you should be eating with Hypothyroidism

Super-foods are considered to be nutrient-rich powerhouses that are beneficial for overall health and well-being. Eating these super-foods may reduce the risk of chronic disease and lengthen your life. Along with essential nutrients, super-foods feed our body the necessary nutrients that our Standard American Diet is lacking.

The Standard American diet in a nutshell is loaded with unhealthy saturated and Trans fats. Our meals are unbalanced, over-sized and loaded with sugar, salt, artificial ingredients and preservatives. We have an abundance of food at our finger tips but yet we are extremely malnourished and mineral deficient. We are literally starving our bodies to death! People are not obtaining the basic nutrients their bodies needs in order to fuel what is needed to perform its proper functions.

We are literally running on empty! There is about 20 million estimated Americans with some type of hypothyroid disorder.

Although your thyroid is small, it produces a hormone that influences every cell, tissue and organ in the body. The thyroid determines the rate in which your body produces the energy from nutrients and oxygen. What if you could start eating foods to feed your thyroid? What if you could start nourishing your body back to health with foods that jump kick your metabolism? Foods that are powerful enough to help you lower your cholesterol, reduce your risk of heart disease and cancer? Are you interested?

I really don't like labeling a certain number of foods as "super" to just 21. There are so many other foods out there that pack a powerhouse punch but if you are affected by hypothyroidism these foods that I have listed will start to feed your body the nutrients that it is lacking. Make sure you eat the color of the rainbow. Fill your plate with a lot of fibrous vegetables that will help you lose weight, stay fuller longer and improve your skin. When you eat fibrous vegetables it passes through your body undigested, keeping your digestive tract running smoothly and helping your bowel movements flush out cholesterol and harmful carcinogens. Fibrous foods are asparagus, green beans, beetroot, cooked broccoli, cooked Brussel sprouts, carrots, celery, cucumber, garlic, lettuce, mushrooms, onions tomatoes and cooked spinach. Many people with hypothyroidism are deficient in Magnesium, B-12, Zinc, Iodine, B2, Vitamin C, Selenium, Vitamin D and Vitamin A.

Blueberries are nutrient dense and are loaded with fiber, vitamin c, vitamin K, manganese, antioxidants, fights cholesterol, lowers blood pressure, fights cancer and boosts brain health.

Pumpkin is loaded with antioxidants, fiber, Vitamin A, Vitamin C, magnesium, potassium , zinc, contains L tryptophan, a chemical compound that triggers feelings of well-being that aid depression and is anti-inflammatory which means it helps with joint health, organ health, stress relief and soft tissue injuries!

Gluten free oatmeal are suitable for a gluten-free diet. People with hypothyroidism typically have a gluten intolerance. Oatmeal with fuel your body, give you fiber, help lower your cholesterol, enhance your immune system and help stabilize your blood sugar.

Free-range or "pastured" organic eggs contain Tryptophan and Tyrosine which is important for the prevention of cardiovascular disease and cancer. They are loaded with all 9 essential amino acids choline, powerful antioxidants and sulfurB12, vitamin A, omega-3 fatty acids, vitamin e, iron, phosphorous, selenium and B2 and B5.

Beans, beans, beans the magical fruit! The more you eat the more you toot! Eating foods that cause gas is the only way for the microbes in the gut to get nutrients. They are full of nutrients, including protein, fiber, slow-burning carbs, antioxidants, vitamins, and minerals. Healthy individual can have up to 18 flatulences per day and be perfectly normal per Purna Kashyap, a gastroenterologist at the Mayo Clinic in Rochester, Minn.

Red bell peppers is an excellent source of vitamin C, vitamin E, manganese, and antioxidant-rich, six different carotenoids (alpha-carotene, beta-carotene, lycopene, lutein, cryptoxanthin and zeaxanthin).

Sardines are rich in omega-3 fatty acids EPA and DHA, which have been found to lower triglycerides and cholesterol levels. Sardines are an excellent source of vitamin D, vitamin b12 and rich in protein, which provides us with amino acids.

Brazil nuts are a very good source of vitamin-E, Vitamin B, thiamin, riboflavin, niacin, pantothenic acid, folates, copper, magnesium, manganese, potassium, calcium, iron, phosphorus, and zinc. Just two Brazil nuts per day can give you the recommended daily allowance of selenium. Most hypothyroidism patients are selenium deficient.

Dark chocolate Cacao not cocoa are two different kinds of chocolate. Once the beans are roasted and processed that they are called cocoa. Most cocoa powders have additives like sweeteners or cocoa butter. The cocoa beans lose much of their nutritional benefits. Cacao is the purest form of chocolate you can eat. It is raw and much less processed than store bought cocoa powder. It's full antioxidants, magnesium, iron, potassium, calcium, zinc, copper and manganese.

Wild salmon is loaded with omega 3 fatty acids, High Quality Protein, Essential Amino Acids, Vitamin A, Vitamin D, Vitamin B6, Vitamin B, Vitamin E, calcium, iron, zinc, magnesium, and phosphorus.

Seaweed contains vitamins A, vitamin C, and calcium and is a natural source of iodine. Iodine deficiency is common with people who have hypothyroidism. Symptoms of being iodine deficient are fatigue, depression, difficulty losing weight and are a higher chance of becoming sick.

Chia seeds contain Zinc, Vitamin B3 (Niacin), Potassium, Vitamin B1 (Thiamine), fiber, protein, magnesium, Vitamin B2, calcium, phosphorus, loaded with Antioxidants, almost all the carbs in chia seeds are fiber, they have more Omega-3 fatty acids than salmon and has been shown to lower LDL cholesterol and triglycerides, increase HDL cholesterol and reduce inflammation

22 Tips To start Naturally Start Healing Your Thyroid

Once you start to address these underlying issues only then can your body can start heal but 1st what are you addressing exactly?

Your body is an awesome design but there is a complex balance between everything. It's like a domino. One thing in your body that is overworked   can cause a major shift in how things operate. Sometimes we have to do a little pruning of the branches, in order for the tree to be healthy again. There is not one size fits all.

See we have to get your thyroid isn't working properly it can wreak havoc on your life. Your thyroid is responsible for so many things. it regulates your metabolism, makes energy, adjusts your mood, helps you sleep, even helps aid in good digestion but your see this is where you come into play. Like anything else in life you get back what you give. Start today following these tips and you will start healing your thyroid naturally.

You have to be in charge of your health.

#1 Find a good holistic practitioner or a doctor who will listen to you and run the proper tests. A practitioner will also start searching for the underlying issues of your hypothyroidism. They will give you advice and solutions to work towards finding the answer. We all are different and make up uniquely. What is my reason for having hypothyroidism might not be your reason.

TSH (Thyroid Stimulating Hormone)

TSH – This is a pituitary hormone that responds to low/high amounts of thyroid hormone that is moving around in your blood stream. In some cases of Hashimoto's and primary hypothyroidism, this lab test will be elevated. In the case of Graves' disease the TSH will be low. People with Hashimoto's and central hypothyroidism may have a normal reading on this test.

Thyroid peroxidase antibodies (TPO Antibodies) & Thyroglobulin Antibodies (TG Antibodies)

Thyroid peroxidase antibodies (TPO Antibodies) and Thyroglobulin Antibodies (TG Antibodies) – People with Hashimoto's will have an elevation of one or both of these antibodies.

Free T3 & Free T4

Free T3 & Free T4 – These tests measure the levels of active thyroid hormone moving around in the body.

Reverse T3

Basic Metabolic Panel

Ferritin level (iron)

So, don't allow your doctor to perform a standard TSH test. Those in itself are simply unreliable. You want to have vitamin panels, hormone panels, candida test, Lyme tests, and adrenal tests too.

#2 Keeping your Blood Sugar in Check

Low GI (glycemic index)/ Low Carb diets are based on the principles of balancing your blood sugar. The reason for keeping your blood sugar in check is to not have your blood sugar and insulin levels to rise to fast and high. This roller coaster of blood sugar highs and lows will activate your stress hormones and are catabolic to our tissues including the gut lining, lungs and brain. Your body is in one of two states throughout the day. You're either in an anabolic state or a catabolic state. If your body is in a constant catabolic state the protective barriers will become worn down over time and it over activates the immune system creating chaos where the body gets confused and attacks itself and wasting away as is the case with Hashimoto's or basically any autoimmune condition. Three things also can contribute to a catabolic state. Not working out smart. Not eating the right food. Not getting enough rest. If you are in a catabolic state you take the change of your body cannibalizing muscle. If you're in an anabolic state is it means that you're exercising correctly, you're eating the right foods and you are getting plenty of rest. Remember you can be creating more cortisol to store in your mid-section by over exercising. You want to stimulate the metabolism, not annihilate it. The easiest way to balance blood sugar and remain in an anabolic state is to eliminate processed carbohydrates and sugar, plan meals around protein and healthy fats then load up your plate with low carb/low GI.

#3 Eat more Nutrient Dense Foods

Think about what you're putting in your body. Either you're fighting disease or feeding disease. You must get a concept of nutrient density. Many of the foods we tend to eat, block nutrients from being absorbed. Gluten, dairy and soy products create inflammation in the digestive tract. In ancient times grains were prepared by soaking, sprouting and fermenting but that tradition in making them been long forgotten with our fast-paced culture. If you have inflammation in the digestive system undigested proteins leak into the blood stream creating a heightened immune reaction that often makes your thyroid issues worse and can lead to a leaky gut which causes other problems.

Olives

Avocado

Cooked Cruciferous vegetables (Limit this to no more than 2x per week)

Fermented foods

Fatty fish (e.g., wild-caught salmon trout, tuna and mackerel.)

Chicken and Turkey (organic hormone & Antibiotic free)

Grass Fed Beef

Leafy greens

Nitrate free bacon

Nuts, such as walnuts and almonds

Seeds, such as pumpkin, chia and flax

Coconut Flour, Almond Flour and hemp seeds

Chia Seeds

Kelp and seaweed

Celtic or Himalayan sea salt

Low carb/ Low-glycemic fruits and vegetables

Coconut oil

Organic butter (preferably Grass fed)

Ghee

Bone Broth

Eggs: Look for pastured or omega-3 whole eggs. (if you don't have a food allergy)

Cheese: Unprocessed cheese (cheddar, goat, cream, blue or mozzarella).

Fish oil (EPA/DHA)

Magnesium

Vitamin B Complex

Vitamin C

Vitamin D3

Zinc

Ancient Nutrition- Bone Broth Collagen Loaded with Bone Broth Co-Factors

#4 AVOID SOY

You must be confused about soy as so much has been said about this little bean. Well, if you have a thyroid condition, it's likely that your hormonal health overall has been compromised. It's best to avoid soy as it elevates the estrogen levels.

Food to avoid: tofu, soymilk, soy lecithin (used as fillers in f.eg veggie burgers), and soy oil.

Fermented soy like miso and tempeh are OK though. Always pick non-GMO (non-genetically modified) and MSG-free miso and tempeh)

#5 FIND OUT WHAT FOOD SENSITIVIES YOU MIGHT HAVE –

It is believed that as much as 70% of our current population has some form of food sensitivities (different from allergies) and the main culprits are:

Gluten

Soy

Dairy

Eggs

Yeast

Fructose

Nuts

Lugumes

How do you know if you have it? Eliminate one food culprit at a time for 2 weeks, see if you feel any better, and then re-introduce it in large amount after the 2 weeks. If symptoms (such as bloating, headaches, fatigue, foggy brain, eczema, acne, etc.) come back, you know the culprit. It's critical to cut out the culprit(s) as it aggravates your immune system.

#6 GETTING ENOUGH IRON– it's said that 60% of people with thyroid conditions are iron deficient. It's best to get a blood test to know for sure but typical symptoms include anemia, cracking of corners of the mouth, inflamed tongue, dizziness, hair loss, brittle nails, fragile bones, sensitivity to cold, depression and confusion. Be generous with food rich in iron: liver (of any animal) and organs, beef, chicken, fish, clams, cooked spinach, lentils and butter beans. Iron is best taken by itself; on an empty stomach but if it irritates your stomach take it with a vitamin C type food. Also when you are taking an iron supplements avoid coffee, tea, calcium rich products, antacids' and soy products this will interfere with the absorption of the iron.

#7 LIMIT YOUR INTAKE OF GOITEROUS FOODS– Goiter is a substance that slows down your thyroid. If you have hypothyroidism: You must limit them. Only eat cooked goiterous foods twice per week.

#8 Supplements and Medication Interactions

When it comes to thyroid medications, it's important for you to know the medications can interact with common nutritional supplements. Calcium supplements have the potential to interfere with proper absorption of your thyroid medications. Wait 4 hours after your thyroid medication before you take anything with calcium in it.

#9 AVOID GLUTEN

Gluten causes an autoimmune reaction. Research has shown a link between wheat allergies and thyroid disease.

#10 START COSUMING COCONUT OIL

Raw, Virgin Coconut oil has been used as just one hypothyroidism natural treatment. Coconut oil is made up of medium chain fatty acids known as medium chain triglyceride's (MCTs), which help with metabolism and weight loss, coconut oil can also raid basal body temperatures – all good news for people suffering from low thyroid function.

#11 NUTRIENT DEFICIENCIES

The most common nutrient deficiencies are Protein, iodine, Magnesium, B-12, Zinc, Iodine, B2, Vitamin C, Selenium, Vitamin D, Vitamin A and iron. Have your doctor run a panel to check for these. The best way to prevent a deficiency is to eat a balanced, real food-based diet that includes nutrient-dense foods (both plants and animals)

#12 DRINK GUT HEALING BROTH

Bone broth is the new green juice. It is full of vital nutrients that will start healing your gut and strengthens your weaken immune system. Most people have a leaky gut and doesn't even know it. Add a pinch of Himalayan sea salt and some kelp flakes for an extra added boost of nutrition. Read here for more information on bone broth and a great easy recipe.

Gut-Healing Vegetable Broth

12 cups filtered water

1 tbsp. coconut oil

1 red onion, peeled and cut in half

1 garlic bulb smashed

1 chili pepper roughly chopped

1 thumb-sized piece of ginger roughly chopped

2 cups of watercress

3-4 cup mixed chopped vegetables and peelings I used carrot peelings, red cabbage, fresh mushrooms, leeks and celery

1/2 cup dried shiitake mushrooms

1/4 of a cup dried wakame seaweed

1 tbsp. peppercorns

2 tbsp. ground turmeric

1 tbsp. organic apple cider vinegar

A bunch of fresh parsley

Simply add everything to a large pot. Bring to a boil then simmer, with the lid on, for about an hour.

Once everything has been cooked down, strain the liquid into a large bowl.

#13 Avoid unnecessary body chemicals

These are commonly found in items like antibacterial soap, deodorant, lotions, and makeup. These things are poisonous. Your skin is the largest organ in the body. Whatever you put on your skin goes into your body. I can't preach this enough. If you can't eat it, then don't apply it to your skin. I understand this might not be 100% doable but every little bit helps your body.

#14 Start Loving YOURSELF Again

All you seem to do is run, run and run! You are exhausted and feel guilty anytime you need to have down time because there are always things that need to be done. So why don't you start to allow yourself to take a day and do nothing. I mean absolutely nothing. WHY? Because your body needs to recharge and stop being ran into the freaking ground. You are not a machine. Start simple like an Epsom salt bath. Get up take a shower and put on more pajama's. Make a movie day.

#15 BE YOUR OWN HEALTH ADVOCATE

Research and study. No one needs you more than yourself. After being diagnosed my priorities were made clearer. I had to start listening to my body, stop taking my health for granted and continuing to research to figure out what I needed to do to "fix me".   A lack of knowledge is a lack of power

#16 Boost your Immunity with Better Gut Health

We are consumed with little fiber and an excess of sugar, salt, and processed foods. Stress, changes in the diet, contaminated food, chlorinated water, and numerous other factors can also alter the bacterial flora in the intestinal tract. When you treat the whole person instead of just treating a disease or symptom, an imbalance in the intestinal tract stands out like an elephant in the room. Read more on Booting your Immunity with better gut health here.

#17 EAT SEA VEGTABLES TWICE PER WEEK

Sea vegetables are a good natural source of iodine to support the thyroid. It's super easy to add start adding some sea veggies into your diet. You can add a piece of kombu to a pot of beans or soup during cooking or sprinkle kelp granules over your salads or add to hot dishes just like you would use salt and make a nori wrap.

#18 BE KIND TO YOUR ADDRENALS

Your adrenals and your thyroid have a strange relationship. They contradict each other all the time. They have a topsy-turvy relationship in which when one goes up, the other goes down. If you are always exhausted you might want to start addressing your adrenals. You can find more information on this topic in my latest book.

#19 Start practicing YOGA

Yoga can stimulate and support the entire endocrine system and not over stress your adrenal gland which can raise your cortisol levels and add fat around your waist.

#20 Up Your Selenium and Zinc

Studies have shown that a severe zinc or selenium deficiencies can cause decreased thyroid hormone levels. Never take zinc on an empty stomach. Brazil nuts are high in both zinc and selenium. Selenium is a micro-nutrient and antioxidant contained in foods like shellfish, cold-water fish, nuts and seeds. the recommended daily intake of this essential mineral is only 70 micrograms and extreme selenium-deficiency is rare, minor to moderate cases are not unheard of. Over time, selenium-deficiency can lead to Hashimoto's disease which causes the immune system to attack the thyroid. Signs to look for include unexplained muscle and joint pain, very dry or brittle hair, and an abundance of white spots on the fingernails.

#21 Avoid all sources of fluoride

As I've mentioned in every one of my books and on blog website. Fluoride suppresses the thyroid and can be your leading cause of hypothyroidism. We all are unique Start drinking filtered water, avoid soft drinks, use fluoride-free toothpaste, use a shower filter, and throw away non-stick cookware. Keep in mind that coffee and tea naturally contain fluoride.

 # 22 Avoid harsh chemicals: You can start making your own natural cleaning supplies cheaply and without the cost of your health. You can google how to make your own cleaning products or purchase my book, **Awareness has Magic**, I have a ton of nontoxic safe alternatives recipes.

You should have a better understanding to why these 6 Things are vital to your health and recovery. I've given you many tools in this book to start working on these 6 area's in your life right now. All I can give you is the blueprint of things you can start doing today to incorporate a healthier you. Taking charge of your health doesn't have to be complicated. The journey has just begun. Each day is filled with the opportunity to make an impact and have that ripple effect with your health. There is no such thing as something for nothing. You have the abundance of good health within your reach.

#1: Immune System

#2: Digestive System

#3: Inflammation

#4: Stress

#5: Start Being Aware

#6 Rule out other causes of your symptoms

   Nutrient deficiencies

  Candida Yeast overgrowth

  Food Allergies

Super Effective Homemade Body-wrap Recipes for Various Body Issues that Work

I am going to share with you the truth about on how to make Super Effective Homemade Body-wrap Recipes for Various Body Issues that Work MADE IN YOUR KITCHEN! These all natural recipes are easy solutions that you can create yourself and avoid unnecessary hormone changing chemicals that are in commercial body wrap brands.

Body wraps are worn to help you shed inches, detox your skin while also hydrating those hard to manage areas. I know the idea of making your own body wraps might not seem to be that glamorous as being in a high-end trendy spa. I will tell you all you need to know and show you the right formulas along with the perfect techniques of making and wearing a homemade body wraps. Follow my instructions while using these 100% organic ingredients and you will see satisfactory results in as little as 7 days!

It's this simple!

Make sure you always start each wrap with a full body skin exfoliation. Next you will apply a thick layer of your chosen combined ingredients is rub it on your body. After that you will wrap up in an organic nontoxic plastic wrap or any other material which will promote blood circulation, boost your immune system, and make you sweat.

Getting the Most Out of Your Homemade Body Wraps

Let's be realistic here. If you want to see the results that you desire you must also do a few things listed below to help you get to your goal. You can't wrap your body and continue following the same old routine that might have given you that unsightly blemish that you want to get rid of. Here are a few body wrap suggestions to help you get that bulge-free body you desire.

1. 100% Organic Ingredients

If you want to see inches come off then you must use 100% organic ingredients only or else you're wasting your time and these cellulite-busting, fat-fighting, skin-glowing, detoxifying recipes won't do you any good.

2. Commercial Brand Body Wrap Kits

Don't be tempted by these premade kits that tend to have harsh hormone changing synthetic chemicals and are made in a lab when you can use these all natural healthy-safe ingredients and get more bang for your buck.

3. Exfoliate, Exfoliate, Exfoliate

Dry brushing before you wrap not only Stimulates Your Lymphatic System, it Exfoliates, Increases Circulation, Reduces Cellulite, reduces Stress, reduces water retention and Improve Digestion and Kidney Function along with being Invigorating. You may even become "addicted" to dry skin brushing because it simply feels so fantastic. Along with glowing and tightening the skin.

"The lymphatic system is responsible for collecting, transporting to the blood, and eliminating the waste our cells produce," "If the lymphatic system is congested, it can lead to a build-up of toxins, causing inflammation and illness. Dry brushing stimulates the lymphatic system as it stimulates and invigorates the skin."

After you exfoliate you take quick steamy hot shower and scrub and buff at that dead, dry, flaky skin to reveal silky soft smoothness. Allow the steam to help open your pores so that your high-quality, organic ingredient body wrap sinks in to the deepest layers of your skin.

How do dry brush? Start at your feet and brush upward towards the heart. Use firm, small strokes upwards, or work in a circular motion. For the stomach, work in a counterclockwise pattern. Harsh exfoliation is never the point; be sure not to press too hard, or use too-stiff of a brush. "Any kind of brushing or exfoliation should be gentle and should never break the skin."

4. Fight Fat with Water

Drinking water makes your skin glow and is important for overall good health because water aids in digestion, circulation, absorption and even excretion. ... And skin cells, like any other cell in the body, are made up of water. Without water, the organs will certainly not function properly or at their best also staying properly hydrated will help shrink your fat cells and remove fat from them.

5. Exercise

Exercise is one of the most important parts of keeping your body at a healthy weight. Your job isn't done once you take off that wrap. Exercise will help you in a battle to shed extra weight if you need to and it lowers the risk of some diseases even if you don't need to lose any weight.

6. Keep at it

If you want this to work, don't try a few sessions, get bored and quit. You should maintain a consistent body wrapping routine and stick to it for permanent results.

7. Be Realistic

Have fun with this. Life is too short to stress and remember that it's a slow and gradual process. So, don't expect overnight results.

8. Use PVC free plastic wrap

The dangers of wrapping your stomach in plastic don't just stop there. Cling wrap used for wrapping the stomach is made from Polyvinyl chloride (PVC), which has been described as one of the most dangerous consumer products. It leaches harmful substances which have been linked to negative effects on the liver, spleen, kidneys, bone formation and body weight. PVC is also linked to cancer. Some wraps are dipped in mineral products, some of which may contain aluminum, which is linked to Alzheimer's. In addition, you may be allergic to some of the ingredients used in the wrap.

9. Use Spa Slender Body Wraps

I really like the Velcro on the ends. No more holding one side and completing a wrap to hold the end in place only to have it pop off. These hold securely and make getting started effortless. If anything, it holds too well. These body wraps are latex free, 6 Inches wide x 15 Feet long (15 feet when stretched), Velcro Closure on Both Ends No Metal Clips, Latex Free, and Durable and most important they are Washable and Reusable.

Tips

Soak every two days in a 1 cup Epsom salt, 1 cup baking soda and 1 cup bentonite clay tub to help flush out the accumulated toxins.

Drink plenty of water before and after using the body wrap to help flush out the toxins from your body. Keep a glass of water handy while you're using the wrap in case you need to hydrate.

Make sure the room you're in while using the wrap is warm. This will prevent the wrap from losing heat too fast, and it will help you to remain warm.

Use twice wrap once a week for about six weeks, then once a month thereafter for maintenance.

Use wrapping cloths specifically designed for use with body wraps or PVC free plastic wrap.

Wrapping your body can be tricky. If you feel comfortable, ask for the help of a friend when it's time to wrap.

#1. Cellulite

The Cellulite Body wrap

Seaweed and clay both act as powerful ingredients in battling cellulite, shifting inches and rejuvenating your body. Here's how you create one of the most effective wraps for cellulite:

What You Need:

1 cup Seaweed Powder

3 tablespoons Almond Oil or Olive Oil or any oil you like

2 cups warm water (or coffee for an extra cellulite-busting kick)

2 drops essential oil (Rosemary, juniper, or fennel)

Method:

Mix all the body wrap ingredients to form a mud-like consistency. Stand in your tub or on newspapers or a large towel to avoid a mess. Start by smearing the paste all over your lower half body.

Now you have two options:

Wrap yourself in plastic, followed by bandages, as plastic increases heat;

Or wrap your lower half in bandages dampened in warm water for hydration.

Both methods work well. Choose what works for you and go with it. Wrap yourself in a blanket and relax for one hour. Remove all seaweed with a warm shower.

#2 – Weight Loss

The Skin-Tight Jeans Body wrap

What You Need:

- 2 cups green tea (or water but green tea helps with weight loss)
- 1 cup bentonite powder (clay)
- 2 drops of a Slim & Sassy (diuretic essential oil)

Method:

Mix all ingredients to form a paste. Do not use a metal bowl as it might react to the clay and draw traces of the metal. Follow the directions of the body wrap described above and do ensure that you take a good shower to remove all traces.

#3. – Detoxification

The Epsom Salts Detox Body wrap

What You Need:

1 cup Epsom salt

4 cups chamomile herbal tea bag steeped water

3 tablespoons almond oil or coconut oil

2-3 drops Rosemary essential oil

Old sheet

Method:

Mix the boiled water that has been cooled to a warm temperature with the salt. Soak an old sheet in the solution. Massage the oil on your body. Wrap yourself in the warm sheet, followed by a plastic to keep it all nicely packed for proper sweating. Spread a blanket and lie on it for an hour to naturally sweat it out.

#4. – Detoxification

The Apple Cider Detox Body wrap

What You Need:

1 cup bentonite powder (clay)

1 cup apple cider vinegar (remember to skin test first, and dilute if necessary with water) chamomile herbal tea bag steeped water

1 cup of water

2-3 drops Slim & Sassy essential oil

Old sheet

Method:

Mix all ingredients to form a paste. Do not use a metal bowl as it might react to the clay and draw traces of the metal. Follow the directions of the bodywrap described above and do ensure that you take a good shower to remove all traces.

#5. – Circulation

The Ginger Clay Bodywrap

What You Need:

2 tbsps. Ginger powder (less for sensitive skin)

5 tbsps. Bentonite clay powder

10 tbsps. Warm water

Method:

Mix up everything by hand or in a blender to form a paste. Smear the paste on the body parts where you want to boost circulation and wrap up with plastic. Rinse off with warm water after 20-40 minutes max. And finish off with a cold rinse.

#6. – Muscle Pain

The Caliente Body wrap

What You Need:

2 tbsps. Cayenne powder (less for sensitive skin)

10 tbsps. White clay

20 tbsps. Warm water

Method:

Make a thick paste of all the ingredients and warm it in the microwave for a few seconds. Apply on the area where it hurts the most and let it sit for 10-12 minutes. Wrap with plastic for more heat and sweat but be careful as the cayenne powder might burn your skin. Shower with warm water.

#7. – Rejuvenating Skin

The Olive Oil Beauty Detox Body wrap

What You Need:

- 2 cups almond or olive oil
- 7-8 drops grapefruit essential oil
- 2-3 drops lavender oil

Method:

Mix up all the oils and pour into a spray or squirt bottle. Spray all over your skin and wrap up in plastic and bandages for a smooth, snug fit. Stay in a warm area for one hour and shower it off with warm water.

Getting on the Right Medication

How do you know if you are on the right type of thyroid medication?

Let's discuss a few important things without it sounding like a foreign unknown language:

There are two forms of thyroid hormone floating around in your body.

1. T4 or Thyroxine - This is the carrier form of thyroid hormone. T4 is a hormone has a role in many of the body functions, including growth and metabolism. There are two kinds of T4 tests: a total T4 test and a free T4 test. A number of drugs can interfere with your T4 levels, so tell your doctor what medications you're taking before a T4 test. T4. Some of your T4 is called free T4. Free T4 doesn't bond well to protein in your blood. Most of the T4 in your body does bond with protein.

2. T3 or Triiodothyronine - This is the active form of thyroid hormone and the majority in your body comes from T4 conversion to T3. T4 can turn into either the active T3 or the inactive reverse T3.

Many doctors give out T4 only medication and hope that your body will have no problem converting the T4 into the active thyroid hormone T3. Sometimes there isn't a problem and T4 medication works perfectly fine.

Contrary to the old ways on the process of shifting the T4 into T3 is constrained by a number of things that affect thyroid overall function which are: Stress, Insulin resistance, Leptin resistance, Prescription medications and Chemical toxins.

Some patients seem to do better on some form of T3 (triiodothyronine) added to their current thyroid medication.

Thyroid medication options:

1. T4 only medications

Synthroid (Levothyroxine), Levoxyl, Tirosint

Synthroid T4 only medication

Levoxyl t4 only medication

Tirosint t4 medication

2. T3 only medications

Cytomel (liothyronine) or Sustained Release T3 (from compounding pharmacy)

liothyronine t3 only medication

3. Combination of T3 and T4 medications

Natural Dessicated Thyroid - Armour Thyroid, Westhroid, Naturethroid, etc.

Combinations of T4 and T3: Cytomel + Synthroid or Combos from compounding pharmacies.

Armour Thyroid compounded T4 and T3

Westhroid combo of T4 and T3 medication

Naturethroid combo t4 and t3 medication

If you are on a T4 only medication (like Synthroid or levothyroxine) and you are still symptomatic, it might benefit you if you add some form of T3. Then again, your medication could be exactly what you need but you're not addressing other issues like for instance your gut health, environmental toxins, eating right, your stress, your sleep or even other medications that you are taking. This isn't a one size fits all fix. You must start working on other area's in your life too. If you want to get better.

Some people do decide to take Natural Dessicated Thyroid (NDT), and other people do require higher amounts of T3 only medication and benefit from taking Cytomel alone or a combination of Cytomel and Synthroid together.

Remember we are all individual's. The type of thyroid medication and the dose you need will depend solely on your own body. Don't assume that if a certain medication worked for Sally it will work for you.

Trial and error, along with blood work, how you feel and paying attention to your symptoms are the best way to find your type of medication and dosage.

 Thyroid Resistance and Reverse T3

Thyroid resistance is a recently new term that means that your cells are resistant to thyroid hormone. Sounds crazy, huh?

Hopefully, I won't make you fall asleep or completely confuse you with this. So here goes.

Your body adapts T4 to the inactive hormone reverse T3. If you have too much reverse T3 in your blood, it will sit on top of the T3 receptor and blocks T3 from entering the cells. Sounds strange doesn't it? Reverse T3 is the "bully" form of the T3 hormone. Blood work will be able to determine if you have higher levels of reverse T3. In which all you have to do to fix this is add more T3 hormone and cut back on your T4 medications.

Your Thyroid Medications isn't working

I need for you to understand that you have to start addressing the root of your hypothyroidism. Just taking thyroid medication is a band-aide solution to putting your hypothyroidism in remission. After you've been diagnosed with Hypothyroidism it means that your thyroid isn't producing the needed thyroid hormone for your body to properly function.

It is important to understand if you have inflammation in your body it will suppress your thyroid hormones and also decreases the responsiveness of thyroid receptors. Look at it this way. You can be dedicated in never missing a dose of thyroid medication and you can also be on the correct dosage as well but if your thyroid cell receptors are blocking the medication to enter due to inflammation that is suppressing your thyroid it's like moving 2 steps forward and 1 step back.

Another thing, if you have inflammation it decreases the conversion of T4 (inactive thyroid hormone) to T3 (active form of thyroid hormone). So if your only taking the synthetic hormone medicines (Synthroid, Unithroid, Levoxyl, etc.) which are only T4, and you have inflammation, it won't work at all because it can't be converted to the active form. To start to restore balance in your body, you must 1st start addressing your hypothyroidism by fixing your immune system and the inflammation that could be raging in your body. Let's not forget that sugar and processed foods can lead to increased inflammation in the body. You must start using more natural remedies while fighting hypothyroidism. The SAD (standard American Diet) is such a poor diet that stresses our bodies more and keeps us lacking the vital nutrients that we need.

Did you know that some medicines can interfere with thyroid hormone production and lead to hypothyroidism, including

◦amiodarone, a heart medicine

◦interferon alpha, a cancer medicine

◦lithium, a bipolar disorder medicine

◦interleukin-2, a kidney cancer medicine

Fermented Foods

A healthy gut plays a significant role in hormone regulation. Having a leaky gut or a lack of probiotic foods lining your intestinal wall can help cause a hormonal imbalance. For most of us, taking a quality probiotic supplement doesn't have any side effects other than higher energy and better digestive health. As a society we have drastically cut back on our consumption of vegetables and of beneficial essential fatty acids (flax, pumpkin, black current seed oil, dark green leafy vegetables, hemp, chia seeds, fish) such as those found in certain fish (including salmon, mackerel, and herring) and flaxseed. We are consume little fiber to no fiber and eat an excess of sugar, salt, and processed foods. Stress, changes in the diet, contaminated food, chlorinated water, and numerous other factors can also alter the bacterial flora in the intestinal tract. When you treat the whole person instead of just treating a disease or symptom, an imbalance in the intestinal tract stands out like an elephant in the room. So to play it safe, I recommend taking a probiotic supplement every. Along with eating fermented foods.

Probiotics are live bacteria and yeasts that are good for your health, especially your digestive system. Probiotics are often called "good" or "helpful" bacteria because they help keep your gut healthy. Probiotics foods include yogurt, kefir,

Kimchi, Sour Pickles (brined in water and sea salt instead of vinegar) Pickle juice is rich in electrolytes, and has been shown to help relieve exercise-induced muscle cramps., Kombucha, kombucha tea ,Fermented meat, fish, and eggs.

Prebiotics foods are brown rice, oatmeal, flax, chia, asparagus, Raw Jerusalem artichokes, leeks, artichokes, garlic, carrots, peas, beans, onions, chicory, jicama, tomatoes, frozen bananas, cherries, apples, pears, oranges, strawberries, cranberries, kiwi, and berries are good sources. Nuts are also a prebiotic source. All these foods that I have listed is hypothyroidism friendly.

The ideal pH for the colon is very slightly acidic, in the 6.7–6.9 range. When there is an imbalance or lack of beneficial bacteria in the colon, the pH is typically more alkaline, around 7.5 or higher. The optimal pH range for gas-producing organisms is slightly alkaline at 7.2–7.3.

When someone starts taking a probiotic or a prebiotic supplement (or eats a prebiotic food), the beneficial microorganisms begin to increase in number. These good bacteria start to ferment more soluble fiber into beneficial products like butyric acid, acetic acid, lactic acid, and propionic acid. These acids provide energy, improve mineral, vitamin, and fat absorption, and help prevent inflammation and cancer. The extra acid also starts to lower the pH in the colon.

Homemade Raw Kombucha Fermented Applesauce

Ingredients

5-6 apples

1/4 cup kombucha - can be plain or flavored.

Instructions

Peel, core, and slice apples. Place in food processor and puree. Add kombucha and puree until you reach desired consistency. Place in sealed mason jar and leave on the counter for 24 hours. Store in fridge. This will stay good for 1 month.

Natural Hormone Balancing

One approach to fixing thyroid issues and hypothyroidism is the use of hormone therapy. You really need to meet with a holistic expert. There are many great holistic and naturopath doctors. Most often, synthetic hormones like Synthroid, Levoxyl, or Levothroid are used, which contain only the T4 hormone and no T3 – two hormones produced by the thyroid gland. Thyroid conditions are serious business. You should always seek a professional who knows how to help you. Our organs and glands like your thyroid, adrenals, pituitary, ovaries, testicles and pancreas regulate most of your hormone production, and if your hormones become even slightly imbalanced it can cause some other serious health issues. Our gut health can also play an important role in hormone regulation. Start loading up on up on rich sources of natural omega-3s like wild fish, flaxseed, chia seeds, walnuts and grass-fed animal products. People don't boost their omega-3 foods intake to balance out the elevated omega-6s they consumed. To many mega-6 foods will cause inflammation and lead to chronic disease. Eating more coconut oil, salmon, grass fed butt like Ghee and avocados will start to provide your body with essential fats that are fundamental building blocks for hormone production. Supplements like digestive enzymes, probiotics, bone broth, kefir, fermented vegetables, and high-fiber foods can start to repair your gut lining, which also can help to balance your hormones. Caffeine will rise your cortisol levels and then it lowers your thyroid hormone levels and basically creates havoc throughout your entire body. Replace your morning coffee with herbal teas. Matcha tea is a great caffeine replacement and is loaded with antioxidants, weight loss benefits, and cancer fighting properties, heart health, brain power, skin health and a good Chlorophyll Source. Last but not least GET OUT IN THE SUN! Free vitamin D, baby. 20 minutes a day is a great way to soak up some that free essential vitamin. On the days where you can't sit out in the sun you can supplement with a good D3 vitamin.

Fluoride blocks iodine receptors

Did you know that fluoride was Once Prescribed as an Anti-Thyroid Drug? Up through the 1950s, doctors in Europe and South America prescribed fluoride to reduce thyroid function in patients with over-active thyroids (hyperthyroidism). (Merck Index 1968). If you haven't already, you should invest in a water filtration system to rid your tap water of fluoride. Do we really know how safe tap water is? Look at the recent events in Flint Michigan! Can you really trust the water companies? Although fluoride concentrations in tap water are relatively low and are considered "safe" for human consumption, it is not. Fluoride has long-term neurological and hormonal affects. Fluoride is not an essential nutrient. It is also that chemical that is commonly found in most toothpaste brands. There is clear evidence that, when ingested at high doses, fluoride causes neurotoxicity. Fluoride also is understood to interfere with the absorption of iodine, possibly leading to an iodine deficiency and ultimately hypothyroidism. To benefit your health, use fluoride free tooth or make your own tooth paste. Get a good water filtration system and purchase a filter for your shower head. We use a British Berkefeld.

Natural Tooth Paste Recipe

Natural Peppermint Toothpaste

1/2 cup coconut oil

3 Tablespoons of baking soda

15 drops of peppermint food grade essential oil

Melt to soften the coconut oil. Mix in other ingredients and stir well. Place your mixture into small glass jar. Allow it to cool completely. When ready to use just dip toothbrush in and scrape small amount onto bristles.

Homemade Coconut Oil Toothpaste Recipe

6 tbsp. coconut oil

6 tbsp. baking soda

15-20 drops of a food grade essential oil (peppermint, cinnamon, grapefruit or lemon taste great)

Melt to soften the coconut oil. Mix in other ingredients and stir well. Place your mixture into small glass jar. Allow it to cool completely. When ready to use just dip toothbrush in and scrape small amount onto bristles.

Keeping your Blood Sugar in Check

Low GI (glycemic index)/ Low Carb diets are based on the principles of balancing your blood sugar. The reason for keeping your blood sugar in check is to not have your blood sugar and insulin levels to rise to fast and high. This roller coaster of blood sugar highs and lows will activate your stress hormones and are catabolic to our tissues including the gut lining, lungs and brain. Your body is in one of two states throughout the day. You're either in an anabolic state or a catabolic state. If your body is in a constant catabolic state the protective barriers will become worn down over time and it over activates the immune system creating chaos where the body gets confused and attacks itself and wasting away as is the case with Hashimoto's or basically any autoimmune condition. Three things also can contribute to a catabolic state. Not working out smart. Not eating the right food. Not getting enough rest. If you are in a catabolic state you take the change of your body cannibalizing muscle. If you're in an anabolic state is it means that you're exercising correctly, you're eating the right foods and you are getting plenty of rest. Remember you can be creating more cortisol to store in your mid-section by over exercising. You want to stimulate the metabolism, not annihilate it. The easiest way to balance blood sugar and remain in an anabolic state is to eliminate processed carbohydrates and sugar, plan meals around protein and healthy fats then load up your plate with low carb/low GI.

Reading Labels

Start reading product labels. You will be surprised where soy, high fructose corn syrup and additives are hiding.

What do we need to do to start healing our hypothyroidism? Let's go over a few things that I've written that are very important things you should know.

The most common allergies and food intolerances are from gluten and dairy (A1 Casein). These proteins are far from simple and can cause a "Leaky Gut" which in return will cause inflammation in your body. The only safe dairy products to consume are from A2 cows, goat milk, sheep milk or nut milks. Gluten creates a havoc in the gut (where the immune system lives) by creating and weakens your immune system.

Start drinking from glass, stainless steel, or BPA free plastic bottles. Bisphenol A (BPA) is found in plastic bottles and can damage your endocrine system and this will have an effect on your thyroid.

Foods, Supplements, and Medication Interactions

When it comes to thyroid medications, it's important for you to know the medications can interact with common nutritional supplements. Calcium supplements have the potential to interfere with proper absorption of your thyroid medications. Wait 4 hours after your thyroid medication before you take anything with calcium in it.

As I've already mentioned in this book that coffee lowers the absorption of your thyroid medication, therefore you need to wait 1 hour before you enjoy that 1st cup. This also goes hand in hand for a fiber supplement.

If you are taking Chromium picolinate, which is marketed for blood sugar control and weight loss, this also interferes with the absorption of your thyroid medications. You should wait four hours between the medications.

Start adding a sprinkle of dulse flakes to your food. Most people with hypothyroidism has low Iodine levels. Kelp and seaweed products can certainly boost your iodine levels. If you start taking a liquid iodine supplement make sure you're under a doctor's care.

Start adding some Milk Thistle, Turmeric, Chlorella, and Cilantro to your smoothies or plate. These food items with help detox harmful metals from your cells and organs.

Start eating more brazil nuts, salmon, sunflower seeds, grass fed beef, mushrooms and onions this is a natural way to get more selenium in your diet.

Get some sun! Vitamin D is often very low with people who have hypothyroidism. You can also start eating more foods like salmon, oysters and sardines. You can add a D3 fermented fish or cod liver supplement. Try to avoid synthetic vitamin D-fortified foods or drinks. Go for the real stuff.

Start eating lower Carbohydrate fruits and veggies. This will lower your body's amount of sugar. Most of us are carb overloaded in this increases estrogen in our body which does negatively affect the thyroid. Add more healthy fats like to help balance your hormones like: coconut oil, coconut milk, avocado, grass-fed beef, wild salmon, chia, flaxseeds, and hemp seeds

Fermented foods are awesome to the belly. They make your gut very happy and from what this book has taught you. A healthy gut is very important to a better digestion and your thyroids health!

Coconut oil

Raw, Virgin Coconut oil has been used as just one hypothyroidism natural treatment. Coconut oil is made up of medium chain fatty acids known as medium chain triglyceride's (MCTs), which help with metabolism and weight loss, coconut oil can also raid basal body temperatures – all good news for people suffering from low thyroid function.

Should I oil pull?

Coconut Oil pulling can really transform your health. Your mouth is the home to millions of bacteria, fungi, viruses and other toxins, the oil acts like a cleanser, pulling out the nasties before they get a chance to spread throughout the body.

 This frees up the immune system, reduces stress, curtails internal inflammation and aids well-being.

An ancient Ayurveda ritual dating back over 3,000 years, oil pulling involves placing a tablespoon of extra virgin organic cold pressed oil (I use coconut oil) into your mouth and then swishing it around for up to 20 minutes, minimum 5 minutes (pulling it between your teeth), before spitting it out. Whatever you do, do not swallow the oil as you will ingest the toxins you are trying to wipe out.

Afterwards requires brushing your teeth with an all-natural fluoride-free toothpaste, and rinsing your mouth out. And you're done! It really is that easy.

Because coconut oil has been shown to:

•Balance Hormones

•Kill Candida

•Improve Digestion

•Moisturize Skin

•Reduce Cellulite

•Decrease Wrinkles and Age Spots

•Balance Blood Sugar and Improve Energy

•Improve Alzheimer's

•Increase HDL and Lower LDL Cholesterol

What Tests Should I Request?

Many cases of thyroid problems can be missed because some won't doctors perform a complete comprehensive thyroid test panel. There are some doctors who will only test your TSH.   Here is a list of tests that you can take to your doctor and request. They will not only test for Hashimoto's and hypothyroidism but other things that might be affecting your health. Be sure to request a copy of your thyroid labs so that you can see them yourself and ensure that they are understood accurately.

1.   TSH (Thyroid Stimulating Hormone)

TSH - This is a pituitary hormone that responds to low/high amounts of thyroid hormone that is moving around in your blood stream. In some cases of Hashimoto's and primary hypothyroidism, this lab test will be elevated. In the case of Graves' disease the TSH will be low. People with Hashimoto's and central hypothyroidism may have a normal reading on this test.

2.   Thyroid peroxidase antibodies (TPO Antibodies) & Thyroglobulin Antibodies (TG Antibodies)

3. Thyroid peroxidase antibodies (TPO Antibodies) and Thyroglobulin Antibodies (TG Antibodies) - People with Hashimoto's will have an elevation of one or both of these antibodies.

4. Free T3 & Free T4

Free T3 & Free T4 - These tests measure the levels of active thyroid hormone moving around in the body.

5. Reverse T3

6. Basic Metabolic Panel

7. Ferritin level (iron)

You also want to check to see if you have any nutrient deficiencies. The most common nutrient deficiencies are Protein, Magnesium, B-12, Zinc, Iodine, B2, Vitamin C, Selenium, Vitamin D, Vitamin A and iron. So, don't allow your doctor to perform a standard TSH test. Those in itself are simply unreliable. You want to have vitamin panels, hormone panels, candida test, Lyme tests, and adrenal tests too. The best way to prevent a deficiency is to eat a balanced, real food-based diet that includes nutrient-dense foods (both plants and animals).

Your morning coffee, Hypothyroidism and your Health

Nothing like that waking up to the smell of coffee. Its gets the juices flowing with that very 1st sip. Its offer you an energetic boost and mental clarity on a feeling that life can go on.

The thyroid gland is such a very important part of the body's regulatory mechanisms; thyroid problems can affect everything in the body from our temperature to appetite to the pulse. Caffeine, a stimulant found in coffee, can affect the thyroid in a number of ways and has an effect on your central nervous system, your digestive tract, and your metabolism.

According to the recent article, in new study from the journal Thyroid people who consume coffee at the time of taking their thyroid medication, we see a 25-57%

drop in T4, one of the thyroid hormones, compared to non-coffee drinkers. This adverse effect persists for up to one hour.

Researchers have also found that for patients taking levothyroxine tablets, absorption is affected by drinking coffee and espresso within an hour of taking the thyroid drugs.

According to "Coffee and Health," by Gerard Debry, in experiments on rats, very high doses of caffeine caused the thyroid gland to enlarge, but at doses of about 300 mg, caffeine in humans did not change levels of thyroid hormones.

What about the benefits? Yes, there are many reliable studies that say coffee is full of antioxidants and polyphenols. However, these same antioxidants and polyphenols can also be found abundantly in many fruits and vegetables.

There are many other reliable studies that show coffee can play a role in the prevention of cancer, diabetes, depression, cirrhosis of the liver, gallstones, etc.

Many coffee drinkers report feeling good for the first two hours (mainly due to a dopamine spike).

(If you just can't give up that morning cup of Joe recommendations by researchers are clear: wait at least sixty minutes after taking levothyroxine before drinking coffee.)

What about decaf you ask?

Many manufacturers use a chemical process to remove caffeine from the coffee beans. The result is less caffeine, but more chemicals. It is the caffeine in the coffee that has the health benefits. Without it, you are left with little benefit.

Increases blood sugar levels

According to this study, caffeine increases blood sugar levels. This is especially dangerous for people with hypoglycemia (or low sugar levels) who feel jittery, shaky, moody and unfocused when hungry. Blood sugar fluctuations cause cortisol spikes, which not only exhaust the adrenals, but also deregulate the immune system. This is highly undesirable for those of us with adrenal fatigue, Hashimoto's or Graves' disease. Such cortisol spikes are also highly inflammatory.

Creates Sugar and Carbohydrate Cravings

As the result of the above, when our blood sugar levels come down, we need an emergency fix to bring them back up. This is why people who drink coffee at breakfast or indulge in sugary and processed breakfasts crave carbs and sugar by 11am or later in the day.

Contributes to acid reflux and damages gut lining

Coffee stimulates the release of gastrin, the main gastric hormone, which speeds up intestinal transit time. Coffee can also stimulate the release of bile (which is why some people run to the bathroom soon after drinking coffee) and digestive enzymes.

In a person with a healthy digestion, this is not a big deal. However, for people with autoimmune conditions, compromised digestion (such as IBS, or "leaky gut"), this can cause further digestive damage to the intestinal lining (source).

Exhausts the adrenals

Coffee stimulates the adrenals to release more cortisol, our stress hormone; this is partly why we experience a wonderful but temporary and unsustainable burst of energy.

What many of us don't realize is that our tired adrenals are often the cause of unexplained weight gain, sleeping problems, feeling emotionally fragile, depression and fatigue. Drinking coffee while experiencing adrenal fatigue is only adding fuel to the fire.

Gluten-Cross Reactive Foods

50% of people with gluten sensitivities also experience cross reactivity with other foods, including casein in milk products, corn, coffee, and almost all grains, because their protein structures are similar. Cyrex Labs provides a test for gluten cross-reactive foods.

Many people report having a similar reaction to coffee as they do to gluten.

Impacts the conversion of T4 to T3 thyroid hormones

Coffee impacts the absorption of levothyroxine (the synthetic thyroid hormone); this is why thyroid patients need to take their hormone replacement pill at least an hour before drinking coffee.

The indirect but important point is that coffee contributes to estrogen dominance, cited above, and estrogen dominance inhibits T4 to T3 conversion.

Highly Inflammatory

Any functional or integrative doctor would say the majority of modern diseases are caused by inflammation – a smoldering and invisible fire found on a cellular level.

This study found that caffeine is a significant contributor to oxidative stress and inflammation in the body. Chronic body pains and aches, fatigue, skin problems, diabetes and autoimmune conditions are just some of the conditions related to inflammation.

Can cause insomnia and poor sleep

This study showed that 400mg of "caffeine taken 6 hours before bedtime has important disruptive [sleep] effects."

There are healthier alternatives to drinking coffee.

Matcha Green Tea Powder

This is a great alternative to coffee. It has caffeine to give you a gentle jolt to wake up, but the caffeine content is nowhere as high as that of coffee, so you won't experience a midday crash and fatigue your adrenals over time. One cup of this wonder tea can keep you going for most of the day.

Natural hypothyroidism Energy Smoothie Recipe

Each ingredient in this smoothie provides necessary nutrients to kick start your day.

•Celery: full of calcium, sodium, copper, magnesium, iron, zinc, potassium. It contains fatty acids and vitamins including vitamin A, C, E, D, B6, B12 and vitamin K as well as thiamine, riboflavin, folic acid and fiber.

•Cucumber: with all its vitamin K, B vitamins, copper, potassium, vitamin C, and manganese, it can help you to avoid nutrient deficiencies that are widespread among those eating a typical American diet.2

•Avocado: full of vitamin K, folate, vitamin C, potassium, vitamin B5, vitamin B6, vitamin E, small amounts of magnesium, manganese, copper, iron, zinc, phosphorous, vitamin A, B1 (thiamine), B2 (riboflavin) and B3 (niacin).

•Romaine: dietary fiber, manganese, potassium, biotin, vitamin B1, copper, iron, and vitamin C. It is also a good source of vitamin B2, omega-3 fatty acids, vitamin B6, phosphorus, chromium, magnesium, calcium, and pantothenic acid.

•Chia seeds: contain lots of fiber, protein, fat: 9 grams (5 of which are Omega-3s), calcium, manganese, magnesium, phosphorus, they also contain a decent amount of zinc, vitamin B3 (niacin), potassium, vitamin B1 (thiamine) and vitamin B2.

•Coconut oil: where do the benefits stop? Check out our full article on the benefits of coconut oil.

•Matcha: adds a boost of slow-releasing, steady caffeine and is packed with antioxidants including the powerful EGCg, fiber, chlorophyll and vitamins. It also provides vitamin C, selenium, chromium, zinc and magnesium.

1 stalk of celery

½ cucumber

½ avocado

1 cup of romaine

1 tablespoon of chia seed

1 tablespoon of coconut oil

1 teaspoon of matcha tea

1.5 cups of unsweetened Almond Milk

Blend and enjoy!

Tazo Organic Chai

This Indian tea is rich in antioxidants and contains a plethora of spices including cardamom, cinnamon, pepper, and ginger that is sure to awaken all your senses in the morning. The smooth creamy flavor actually makes you feel like you are sipping a cup of coffee, but without all the extra caffeine.

Warm Water with Lemon

This is a great way to rehydrate and alkalinize your body and perk up after sleep. It also detoxifies the liver and helps get your bowels going. This really should be the first thing everyone sips in the morning.

Garden of Life RAW Organic Protein Vanilla

Who doesn't enjoy a yummy protein smoothie? It is a terrific way to load up with energy and nutrition. Use almond, soy, or coconut milks and your choice of a good quality protein powder. Throw in some bananas and berries which add heaps of extra minerals, vitamins, and antioxidants that are sure to fill you up and get you going for the grueling day ahead.

Vita Coco Coconut Water

Coconut water is Mother Nature's perfect drink. It has an abundance of electrolytes and minerals while being low in fat and sugar. This is the best alternative to an energy or sports drink, and can really give you a burst of energy in the morning.

Quinoa Milk

Suzie's Quinoa Milk - Vanilla

 This protein-rich natural energy drink may soon make its way into the stores...be prepared almond and soy and coconut milks...it's the next big health thing! Quinoa (pronounced keen-WAH), is a gluten-free, alkaline-forming, high-protein grain that has tremendous health benefits. Click on this link to read more of the healthy benefits!

Quinoa milk can be made from scratch, at home.

Consumers of quinoa milk do not need acreage or a cow to make this refreshment. The ingredients necessary to create quinoa milk can be purchased at a local health food store. The recipe is simple and cost, affordable. Here's a recipe from OmNomNally.com:

Ingredients

1 cup quinoa grain

2 cups + 5 – 6 cups water

1 tsp vanilla extract

1 tsp ground cinnamon

Instructions

Soak quinoa overnight in water and drain on the day of cooking or rinse quinoa in a mesh strainer under running water to remove the bitter saponins. Cook 1 cup of quinoa with 2 cups of water. Add cooked quinoa to blender with 2 cups of water. Blend on high until smooth. Add water to the desired consistency, blending the mixture after each addition. Up to 6 cups total of water may be needed for the consistency of store-bought non-dairy milks. Add vanilla extract and cinnamon and agave if using. Pour milk into nut milk bag, hold over a bowl or large jug. Massage contents until all liquid has passed through the material – leaving only the 'pulp' behind

Kombucha Tea

Yogi Tea Green Tea Kombucha Organic - You've probably heard about this one but don't know too much about it. Kombucha is a type of yeast. When you ferment it with tea, sugar, and other flavors or ingredients you make Kombucha tea. While the benefits of Kombucha are debated, many claim that it is useful for treating memory loss, regulating bowel movements, preventing cancer, helping with high blood pressure, and more.

Guayaki Yerba Mate Organic Tea

Yerba mate is the good alternative to coffee for those who can't start the day without a cup o' caffeine. Providing the same buzz that coffee gives, Yerba Mate is preferred by many as it's packed with nutrients, too. Mate is made from the naturally caffeinated leaves of the celebrated South American rainforest holly tree. It is widely known for not having the heavy "crash" that coffee can bring. Another benefit of Yerba Mate is that it can be prepared and consumed in a variety of ways—hot, cold, with honey, in a tea infuser, in a French press, or even in a traditional coffee machine.

Sparkling Water

Sparkling water can be a refreshing alternative to both coffee and water. Especially when flavored with natural, sugar-free, fruit extracts, sparkling water is delicious and hydrating.

Hot Apple Cider

Hot apple cider's sweet tanginess offers its own unique pick-me-up in lieu of caffeine, and its soothing warmth is just as satisfying as that of coffee on a cold fall or winter morning.

Turmeric Tea

Turmeric is highly anti-inflammatory, and this golden turmeric tea recipe is sure to help heal your body from a number of inflammatory health conditions. Turmeric can help detoxify the liver and protect cell damage caused due to environmental pollutants, attack from free radicals. Research has found that turmeric extracts can lower blood cholesterol levels – especially LDL 'bad' cholesterol. It has lipid lowering properties. This can reduce cholesterol levels and benefit weight loss by reducing adipose tissue weight gain.

This rich creamy and lightly sweet beverage is something you're sure to enjoy!

Turmeric Tea Recipe

Total Time: 5 minutes

Serves: 2

Ingredients:

- 1 cup coconut milk

- 1 cup water

- 1 tbsp ghee

- 1 tbsp honey

- 1 tsp Turmeric (powder or grated root)

Directions:

1. Pour coconut milk and water into the saucepan and warm for 2 minutes

2. Add in butter, raw honey and turmeric powder for another 2 minutes

3. Stir and pour into glasses.

You have to exercise caution when combining it with medications or supplements taken to slow down blood clotting. Turmeric supplements must be stopped two weeks prior to a surgery.

It must not be consumed by diabetic patients, those with gallbladder problems and pregnant and breastfeeding women. Always consult your doctor about the right dosage to consume for a specific medical condition

The Lymphatic System and Your Health

The lymphatic system is your body's natural detox system that is connected as part of your immune system and it is a complex drainage or "sewer" system that consists of glands, lymph nodes, the spleen, thymus gland, and tonsils. Many of us never realize just how important your lymphatic system is nor the fact that it plays one of the largest roles in our bodies by cleansing nearly every bodily cell by removing toxins, metabolic waste and so more. It's also cleanses our cells by absorbing excess fluids, fats, and toxins from our tissues. This waste is pushed into our blood stream where it can eventually be filtered out by the liver and kidneys. Not only is your lymphatic system responsible for flushing out the waste material of the body but it is also responsible for distributing nutrients to each and every part of our body.

When you are living with a nagging health issue like hypothyroidism or Hashimoto's it can be quite trying and you could be doing everything right it seems but yet you are still unable to begin to heal. Did you know that having a clogged lymphatic system could be halting your thyroid from healing? Each Day our bodies are bombarded with a toxic burden of chemicals, we are not feeding our bodies the proper nutrients, we are nutritional deficient, and little to no activity & these are some of the reasons why our system is becoming increasingly polluted. If you have a clogged lymphatic system it won't allow your body to circulate the fluids and eliminate toxic waste buildup which can decrease the body's immune function. This can also increase swelling, inflammation and pain along with the possibility of welcoming other diseases and disorders.

If your lymphatic system is clogged with toxins, and you're trying to cleanse it with the methods in this article, it's important to try to stay away from more toxins! It would be silly to take Motrin for a stone stuck in your shoe when all you had to do was pluck it out. So why not on this journey go ahead and address the issue at hand. Just like I will describe the need for to you to be drinking filtered water, you can't expect your lymphatic system to cleanse if you continue to expose yourself to daily toxins. We all understand that toxins are all around us— from the foods we eat, to the products we use and to the air we breathe. Unfortunately toxins are all around us. It's important to look at your own life carefully to determine where toxins may be the biggest problem and start adjusting your life where needed.

Most often than none, it's unrealistic for any lifestyle change to happen overnight. It does take practice but with practice does come change. Don't allow the bigger picture to discourage you. Every small thing you change to better your health will pay off in the end. It's the small steps that can make a big difference. Start by looking at your life and evaluating the toxins you may regularly come in contact with, understand what must take priority, and replace with these alternative options that I have listed in this article.

(Remember, we each have our own perception of our own realities although we have each walked a different path therefore step out on faith and know that today is the DAY that you begin your journey to a better you. Namaste, Audrey)

How do you know if your lymphatic system is clogged?

There are many ways that your body gives you signs to let you know that your lymphatic fluid is not moving effectively and that the toxins are building up in your body.

Bloating

Swelling in your fingers/rings fitting more tightly

Brain fog

Digestive issues

Parasites

Depression

Sinus infections

Skin problems/dry and or itchy skin

Enlarged lymph nodes

Chronic fatigue

Feeling sore or stiff when you wake up in the morning

Unexplained injuries

Excess weight

Cold hands and feet

Constipation

Worsened allergies

Food sensitivities

Increased colds and flu

Unfortunately, due to our chemical overload, nutritional deficiencies, and less exercise we have allowed our system to become stagnant and polluted. Here are a few things that can happen to your body if your lymphatic system is clogged and needs a serious cleanse:

Skin conditions

Arthritis

Unexplained injuries

Excess weight or cellulite

Headaches

Chronic fatigue

Sinus infections

Digestive disorders

Enlarged lymph nodes

How can I unclog my lymphatic system?

1. Dry Brushing*

Dry brushing is my most favorite way to start each morning. It's very fast to do (takes about 5 minutes) and when you dry brush, your skin becomes invigorated.

Here's why dry brushing is so good for you:

It starts off by shedding the dead skin cells and encourages new cell renewal. Also it relaxes your nervous system. When you dry brush you stimulate the vascular blood circulation and this allows lymphatic drainage to begin. The circulation motion buffs and smooths your skin to making it appear healthier. Don't worry about it feeling odd at first you will get used to it after a few times. Those bristles will start to feel calming while it is refreshing your nervous system, improving nutrient absorption, removing toxins and improving the blood circulation.

Simple steps to dry brushing at home:

Buy a good Dry Brush

Make sure your skin is dry (best to do this before your bath or shower)

Begin from bottom and move upwards. You'll use gentle circular motions or longer smoother strokes or a combination of both.

Always start at your ankles and move toward your heart. Make sure to move the brush in the same direction.

When you get to your back, brush from the neck down instead, toward your lower back.

Be careful with sensitive skin and never brush over sores, sun burned areas or areas with skin cancer.

2. Oil Pulling*

What is oil pulling? Well, it's an ancient Ayurvedic remedy that was used to cleanse the body and enhance oral health. It's helps the body detoxification process and oil pulling helps remove bacteria, parasites and other toxins from your teeth and mucus membranes. It also reduces inflammation in your gums.

How do you do it?

Well, it's actually quite simple. Upon awaking, before eating or drinking anything, take about a tablespoon of organic, virgin, cold pressed, unrefined coconut oil and swish it around in your mouth for 10-20 minutes. I swish it like mouthwash by pulling it through my teeth and over every part in my mouth. After you're finished swishing it, spit out the oil (it will be frothy and pretty gross looking) and next gargle your mouth with mouth out with warm purified water or warm salt-water. Then drink a full 8 oz. drink a glass of water with half of a freshly squeezed lemon.

How it works?

Basically the oil does is mixes with your saliva and this activates enzymes which draw toxins that is in your blood. The fat in the oil helps extract these toxins from your mouth. As the oil absorbs toxins, it becomes whiter, thicker and frothier.

3. Exercise*

Any form of exercise and movement is needed. You see, your circulatory system has your heart to pump blood throughout your body but your lymphatic system doesn't has a "pump" and it is entirely dependent on the movement of your muscles. Walking and yoga are also fantastic ways to get that lymphatic fluid to drain.

It's best to start slow on the exercise and work your way up but be consistent. Think of the tortoise rather than the hare in the beginning and as you get more energy you can exercise longer and harder if you prefer.

4. Lymphatic Drainage Massage*

A lymphatic drainage massage is one easiest way to detoxify that lymph system. Always use a skilled practitioner to stimulate circulation and drain fat, fluids, toxins, and other waste products away from your cells for proper elimination. Acupuncture is another great way to help you with detoxing your lymph system. It's an ancient and effective TCM treatment, also helps opens up the pathways (meridians) in your body by stimulating lymph flow.

5. Rebounding*

Rebounding is one of the easiest and simplest ways to get the blood pumping around those lymph nodes. Rebounding is the practice of jumping on a small trampoline for ten to thirty minutes. This gets the blood flowing while stimulating the circulation of blood throughout the body. If you have Kidney issues this might not be for you. Rebounding can be hard on your kidneys by putting a lot of pressure on them and your body might not be able to handle the extra release of toxins.

6. Organic Apple Cider Vinegar*

OACV helps to break down mucus in your body. It also has been shown to kill various pathogens and bacteria. You will also get the added benefit of it helping improve your blood sugar levels.

7. Inversion Table*

An inversion table is a padded table that allows you to lay upside down while strapped in by your feet. The inversion helps to decompress the joints in the body and stimulates the lymphatic and circulatory system. This allows blood and oxygen to the tissues, which helps to clear out the muscles of toxic build-up. By inverting, gravity works with, not against, the body, encouraging the movement of the lymph system.

8. Meditation*

Start your day out with meditation, deep breathing and a grateful heart. There are many people who weren't able to wake up and live another day. I can't even begin to express the importance of the power of meditation has over the body. It's been proven to lower your levels of cortisol which is also known as the stress hormone. Deep breathing, from your diaphragm, increases oxygen levels and naturally detoxes your body. Breath is life and you can take a breather anywhere, anytime and refocus. I like to start my day off listening to mediation music to clear my head while I have my legs up against the wall using this yoga pose.

Legs up the wall pose will not only help with your thyroid functions but it also relieves back pain, helps with insomnia, improves posture, helps with anxiety, naturally adjusts your spine, improves your digestion and it starts a lymphatic circulation. Your lymphatic system doesn't have a pump and relies on our movements and gravity to circulate lymph fluid where the toxins in this fluid can be eliminated from your body. If we sit all day the lymph fluid becomes stagnant and start to collect toxins. By simply reversing the flow of gravity in your legs, you begin to circulate the lymphatic fluid and encourage the body to start the elimination of toxins. Dry brushing also will simulate the lymphatic system and improve skin tone.

9. Lemon Water*

Warm lemon water helps to stimulate the lymphatic system by helping remove the toxins accumulated in the lymph glands, colon, and bladder. The vitamin C in the warm lemon water help to cleanse the liver and helps to hydrate your lymphatic system. Some cases of lymph congestion is dehydration. Clean Filtered Water and only water can adequately re-hydrate the body. A Lemon is also an alkaline fruit that will help to mineralize the body and your lymph system.

10. Enzymes*

Lymphatic cleaning enzymes were first formulated by Dr. Edward Howell (the deceased author of Enzyme Nutrition), with the purpose of digesting away years of accumulation of these large mucoprotein particles or starch-protein conjugates in the intercellular spaces. Digestive enzymes relieve the workload on the pancreas, and free up other reserve enzymes that are needed elsewhere for your body.

Enzymes are produced by the body to help break down the food we eat and they also assist in helping the body to clear toxic-waste buildup in the lymph and in the blood. If you use a proteolytic enzymes between meals will help to "digest" or breakdown organic debris that are moving through the circulatory and lymph systems, while increasing the lymphatic flow. They also help to lighten the load of allergy-like compounds whose only job is to free up your immune system from these traveling bandits. Never take protein digesting enzymes (protease) during pregnancy, high doses of proteases can thin the blood and if you have gastric or duodenal ulcers, gastritis, or suffer irritation or burning sensations in the stomach, stop taking the enzymes and contact your healthcare practitioner. You should always eat food with protease enzymes rather than taking Enzymes on their own.

11. Eat Raw Foods*

Raw foods help to neutralize harmful pathogens and lessening the burden on the lymph system. Raw foods are alkaline and have higher levels of naturally occurring enzymes that assist in breaking down toxic buildups, encourage the removal of harmful substances in the body and is a great way to help begin the process of flushing out the lymph system. The key is to eat these raw fruits in the am on a empty stomach where the acids and enzymes in the fruit have the best lymphatic draining and stimulating effects. Lemon, lime and grapefruit are wonderful in helping begin the digestive detoxification. Food grade Lemon, lime and grapefruit essential oils work well too just add a few drops to your water throughout the day. All red fruits berries, beets, pomegranates, cranberries, cherries, greens, seaweeds, spirulina, hemp seeds, flax seeds, turmeric, ginger, cinnamon, cardamom and black pepper.

Morning Smoothie

1/2 of a peeled lemon, lime or grapefruit

1 cup of spinach or romaine lettuce (if you have thyroid issue go with the romaine)

1/4 teaspoon of cinnamon

Knob of freshly peeled ginger

1/4 cup of red berry of your choice

1 tablespoon of flax-seed oil

Dash of pepper

Dash of turmeric

1/2 teaspoon of dulse flakes(optional)

16oz. of filtered water

Blend until smooth, pour over ice and drink with a straw. This is very filling too!

12. Always Choose Organic*

Foods that are not organic grown have been sprayed with pesticides, herbicides, insecticides and fungicides and could possibly be genetically modified. This can add to the toxic build up on your lymph nodes.

13. An infrared sauna*

It's great to sweat. Sweating is the body's natural way to release toxins in your system. The sweat excreted through your skin can help release the toxic burden on your lymphatic system.

14. Hot and cold showers*

I understand no one likes taking cold showers but this will greatly benefit the lymphatic system. The hot water helps dilate the blood vessels, and the cold contracts them, creating a "pump" action that helps force fluid that may be stagnant in the system. As I've explained your lymph system has no central pump of its own. This will help to stimulate the flow of your blood and encourage circulation by the expanding and contracting blood vessels. If you are pregnant or have a heart condition always check with your health care provider before attempting this method.

15. Drink equate amounts of clean water*

You've heard it before water is life! Make sure you are drinking filtered water and not adding to your toxic burden by ingesting easily absorbed toxins often present in water such as fluoride, chlorine, VOC's, and more. You can safely consume up to half your body weight in ounces of water a day (160 lbs = 80 ounces of water). I love my Berkey Water Tank!

16. Eating clean*
I mentioned raw foods now let's talk about eating clean whole nutrient rich foods. Start reading label. If you must eat prepacked foods always look for foods that have a short ingredient list and things that are recognizable as actual food. Various chemicals are added like sugars, questionable oils, and sodium and so on. Always avoid soy and if soy is listed as an ingredient. Soy comes in all varieties and are highly processed, high in refined starches, heated oils and again added sugar, salt and low in nutrients and fiber. Oh let's not fail to mention that soy mimics your hormones and plays a very sneaky trick on your endocrine system. Eating clean and mostly raw food that is rooted in produce is

the first step to promoting a healthy lymph flow. These listed are particularly cleansing foods for the lymphatic system:

Dark leafy greens

Fruits in the Low Glycemic index Chart

Garlic

Ground flaxseed

Seaweed

Algae (chlorella, spirulina)

Chia

Avocados

Cranberries

Walnuts

Brazil nuts

Almonds

17. Avoiding Food Allergens*

Many people are unaware that certain foods are actually working against their bodies. You should see a specialist and be tested to ensure you have no food allergies. Your lymphatic system can also be affected by your gut. If your gut is inflamed and not healed this is taxing on your immune system which in return is taxing on your lymphatic system. Consider adding prebiotics and probiotics to help support gut health along with eating properly and avoiding these common food allergens.

Common food allergens that can contribute to an inflamed gut are:

Nightshades

Eggs

Grains (gluten)

Dairy

Lugumes

18. Our words have power*

Our words have power and if we are constantly saying negative things to ourselves or thinking negative thoughts it will eventually begin to affect our body. What comes out of your mouth, goes into your ear & your brain absorbs it. Always be positive and don't allow problems to dwell. The glass is always half full and there is someone who wants what you have. You are a blessing to someone.

19. Adaptogen Herbs

There are numerous herbs have been shown to support the lymphatic system. Some of these herbs include dandelion root, passion flower, nettle leaf, fenugreek, and manjistha. I've taken Echinacea and cayenne pepper together with a healthy fat daily while I was cleansing my lymph nodes. Adaptogen herbs are in a unique class of healing plants that promote hormone balance and also help to protect the body from a wide variety of diseases, including those that are caused by stress. These herbs also boost your immune functions. Research shows that other various adapotogens — such as ashwagandha, medicinal mushrooms, rhodiola and holy basil. Holy basil has been proven to help regulate cortisol levels, protect your organs and tissues against chemical stress from pollutants and the burden of heavy metals, which are other factors that can lead to hormone imbalance, a stagnant lymph system and sickness.

20. Under arm deodorant

Deodorant and antiperspirants impair the underarm lymph nodes. Aluminum-based compounds are the active ingredients in antiperspirants. Sweating is a necessity in life. There are roughly three million sweat glands pumping out as much as 14 liters/ 3 gallons of water a day. Sweat, as stinky and uncomfortable as it can be at times, is a natural and healthy part of life, helping to cool the body, release toxins and helps to maintain normal body temperatures. Sweat isn't inherently stinky either. In fact, it's nearly odorless. The stench comes from bacteria that break down from one of two types of sweat on your skin. Deodorant advertisers have done a pretty neat job of convincing us that we're disgustingly smelly people who in fact need to be refined and save our stinky selves by their products. We've been wonderfully brainwashed into thinking sweating is a bad thing. Sweating from the heat, sweating from exercise, and sweating from stress are all different, chemically speaking. Stress sweat smells the worst. That's because smelly sweat, is only produced by one of the two types of sweat glands called the apocrine glands, which are usually in areas with lots of hair—like our armpits, the groin area, and scalp. The odor is the result of the bacteria that break down the sweat once it's released onto your skin. **Fun fact: While women have more sweat glands than men, men's sweat glands**

Produce more sweat. Commercial deodorants are something you truly need to purge out of your life. Aluminum-based antiperspirants may increase the risk for breast cancer, Alzheimer's disease & Kidney Disease (Scientists noticed that dialysis patients who had these high aluminum levels were more likely to develop dementia too.)

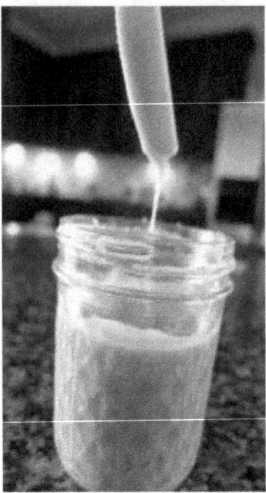

Ingredients

1/2 c. baking soda

1/2 c. arrowroot powder or ½ cup of cornstarch

5 tbsp. unrefined virgin coconut oil

10 drops of grapefruit essential oil or lavender essential oil

You can pick your favorite scent. I like lavender or grapefruit.

Empty deodorant stick or Mason jar

Directions

Mix baking soda and arrowroot together.

Melt your coconut oil in the microwave in a microwave safe bowl.

Mix all ingredients the baking soda and arrowroot powder with the oil, Pour into clean small Mason jar,(or your empty stick container) add your essential oil to the Mason jar or the empty stick container, using a wooden Popsicle stick , give it a good stir to mix everything. Close you're the lid. Once you mix that essential oil in the bowl, it can only be used for the purpose of making your deodorant. Everything you've used is edible except the essential oils.

This will take roughly 24 hours to set. It will thicken up. I use my finger to scrape what I need out of the Mason jar and scoop it across my underarm. This will last you for a good 6 months!

You can also find more great recipes along with this one in my book, AWARENESS HAS MAGIC.

21. Pharmaceutical Drugs*

You really need to do research on your medications. Some medications have a negative effect on your body especially your lymph system.

https://www.lymphnet.org/membersOnly/dl/reprint/Vol_24/Vol_24-N4_Drugs_LE.pdf

22. Personal care products*

Personal care products loaded with parabens, petroleum, and phthalates. Did you know that products we use every day may contain toxic chemicals and has been linked to women's health issues? They are hidden endocrine disruptors and are very tricky chemicals that play havoc on our bodies. "We are all routinely exposed to endocrine disruptors, and this has the potential to significantly harm the health of our youth," said Renee Sharp, EWG's director of research. "It's important to do what we can to avoid them, but at the same time we can't shop our way out of the problem. We need to have a real chemical policy reform." The longer the length of ingredients on your food label means how much more unhealthy it is for you to consume. When an item contains a host of ingredients that most likely you can't even pronounce or remember to spell you can bet your lucky dollar that the natural nutrients are long gone. These highly processed frank n foods are very difficult for the body to break down and some of the chemicals will become stored in your body. Click on this link to see what you should avoid.

You can also find many great DIY personal care recipes alternatives in my book, AWARENESS HAS MAGIC.

Here are three recipes from my book **AWARENESS HAS MAGIC.**

Lemon Cream Body Butter

6 Tablespoons coconut oil

¼ cup cocoa butter

1 Tablespoon vitamin E oil

3 drops of Lemon essential oil or 3 drops of your favorite essential oil

Over low heat in a double boiler, put the coconut oil and cocoa butter in a bowl. When it has almost completely melted, remove from the heat and add the vitamin E oil and essential oil. Allow the mixture to cool until it solidifies. Lastly mix the body butter vigorously with a spatula, and then transfer it to a mason jar with a sealable lid. Date and label your product. If you don't care for the lemon essential oil, use whatever smells best to you. This is your journey not mine I am only here to help guide you.

Homemade Shaving Cream

1 cup shea butter

1 cup virgin coconut oil

3 Tablespoons vitamin E oil

3 Tablespoons sweet almond oil or olive oil or jojoba oil

3 Tablespoons Dr. Bonners Liquid Castile Soap

30 drops of lavender essential oil (optional)

30 drops of lemon essential oil (optional)

I like to use an electric mixer, mixing all ingredients until stiff peaks are formed (approximately 2-3 minutes). Store in a mason jar with a sealable lid.

Mosquito Repellent

15 drops of lavender

4 tbsp. of vanilla extract

1/4 cup freshly squeezed lemon juice

Place all these ingredients in a 16oz then fill with water.

23. Household chemicals*

Did you know that it takes 26 seconds for the chemicals to enter into your bloodstream?

The real reality is we are damaging our DNA and we are changing our genetic makeup for future generations. There was a study a few years back that said the umbilical cord of an average American baby has over 200 known chemicals in it. Eighty percent of the common chemicals that are used daily in this country, we know almost nothing about. Our children are being born toxic and we have no idea if these toxins are already doing some sort of damage their brains, their immune system, their reproductive system, and any other developing organs. Are we unknowingly setting ourselves up for failure in the womb, even before birth?

Scientists and researchers are concerned that many of these chemicals may be carcinogenic or wreak havoc with our hormones, our body's regulating system.

Most products have a warning label that is typed in bold "Keep Out of Reach of Children". As consumers, we believe that if our children don't ingest these products they will not be harmed by them. This can be far from the truth. Think about other common methods of exposure are through the skin and our respiratory tract. WE are along with our children are often in contact with the chemical residues housecleaning products do leave behind, by crawling, lying and sitting on the freshly cleaned floor.

Scientists at Norway's University of Bergen tracked 6,000 people, with an average age of 34 at the time of enrollment in the study, who used the cleaning products over a period of two decades, according to the research published in the American Thoracic Society's American Journal of Respiratory and Critical Care Medicine.

These chemicals can chemicals bind together.

Exposure to phthalates has been associated with lower IQ levels.

These chemicals can also be found in the shampoos, conditioners, body sprays, hair sprays, perfumes, make up, cleaning supplies, colognes, soap and nail polish that we use.

The results follow a study by French scientists in September 2017 that found nurses who used disinfectants to clean surfaces at least once a week had a 24 percent to 32 percent increased risk of developing lung disease.

Scientists and researchers are concerned that many of these chemicals may be carcinogenic or wreak havoc with our hormones, our body's regulating system.

It's not enough to be aware of all the outdoor chemicals that we are exposed to everyday but inside our homes we can have more power and control. We have to be more aware about using chemical cleaners, paints, glues, body lotions, toothpastes, underarm deodorants, hair products and pesticides. Instead start to begin to use products that don't pollute our very own bodies. We must read labels, make our own products and do our own research. I can't stress this enough. We must take a stand for our health. Stop using commercial products that are laced with unknown and harmful body damaging products

You can reduce your exposure to them by eating organic foods, making your own cleaning chemicals and using alternative pest control methods.

You can also find many great recipes for alternative cleaning solutions in my book **AWARENESS HAS MAGIC.**

Here are two recipes from my book **AWARENESS HAS MAGIC**.

Vanilla grapefruit linen spray

2-1/2 cups filtered water

3 drops pink grapefruit essential oil

2 drops vanilla essential oil

1/4 cup vodka

The vodka helps the water dry quickly after you spray it on your linens. Theses essential oils that are used create a beautifully fresh vanilla grapefruit scent that is perfect for a summer pick me up. This spray is very versatile. It can be used on clothing, fabric furniture, or even as a quick air freshener.

If the vodka smell is slightly strong just add another drop or two of essential oil.

Always shake the bottle be before spraying on your linen.

Tub & Tile Cleaner

1 /4 cup baking soda

1/4 cup lemon juice

Or 10 drops of lemon essential oil

3 Tablespoons Epsom salt

3 Tablespoons Sal Suds or Castile liquid soap

1/2 cup white vinegar

Pour the vinegar into the bottle, followed by the baking soda and Epsom salt. Shake the bottle to combine the ingredients. Add the Sal suds gently shaking the bottle to combine. Mix all ingredients in a bottle with a sealable lid.

Scrub and then rinse with water and wet clean rag.

Throughout my latest book, you will find useful, informative and easy to understand recipes for your mind, body and spirit. When I started writing this book, I wanted to introduce you to the idea of a cleaner less toxic world and for you to learn just how simply easy it is for you to start creating your own cleaning recipes throughout your home but this book has transformed into so much more than just a book full of all natural DIY recipes.

This book will enlighten you and help you have a deeper understanding of not only why you should be more aware but how to be more aware. **AWARENESS HAS MAGIC.**

Did You Know That Your Body Has its Very Own Personal Food Code?

There is so much information overload that most women are confused as to where to start to begin creating a healthy lifestyle balance. Perhaps one of the biggest misconceptions is the ambivalence of it all. We all get super busy in this thing called life. Sometimes we lose a little piece of ourselves traveling back in fourth.

How many times this week have you said to yourself, "If my life wasn't so busy, I would be able to start exercising" or" Why did I eat that extra cookie?" or" its 3a.m. "why can't I sleep?!" Or" Why am I so exhausted?"

Frankly, life is one big tug a war between feeling completely insane to the creativity at it all.

Why do we allow ourselves to become Stressed Out, Overwhelmed, and Totally Exhausted and continue to carry around those extra ungodly pounds that we dreadfully despise? After 5 years of carrying that excess weight, I am here to tell you, from one female to another, you can't technically call it baby weight gain any longer.

Have you ever wondered why people respond differently to losing weight?

In the last fifty years what has changed in our society? We have the same predisposition genetics as our grandparents. We are unique and come in all different shapes, sizes, race, religions and greed.

We can't blame is all on genetics being unhealthy solely on the DNA that was passed down to us. Everyone's genetic makeup is different. It's like your fingerprints.

In school, I was always that girl who was tall, skinny, freckled faced, wavy blonde hair with a flat chest and a flat butt. I remember being plagued at school for being too skinny. Having no shape. Tormented about my freckles. While other school mates were well endowed with large boobs, hippy hips and a nice rounder booty. Our metabolisms certainly dictate how we use energy and our genetics can dictate how we are shaped but what has started to interests me more-so lately is why we store fat on certain areas of our bodies when others don't.

These questions have confused and frustrated people and health care practitioners for decades. But why is it so confusing? One thing we have learned is each of us are unique and have our very own biochemistry that sets us apart from everyone else. Although we might share the same common traits and perhaps the same overlapping metabolic tendencies. We can't continue to say that one-size-fits-all when it comes to our very own unique body chemistry. There are over 7 billion people on this planet and we come in all different shapes, colors and sizes. With this being said wouldn't you think the one-size-fits-all- approach to losing weight wouldn't work since we are we are all unique. With this all being said wouldn't you think that we all have our very own personal food code too?

Finding Your Food Code

Finding your food code won't be as easy as it sounds. Quite frankly you will have to put some elbow grease into this but it's not unattainable. How we live from day to day is completely different on every spectrum across the board. One thing I do know for-sure is that every single day no matter who we are or where we live our bodies are bombarded with a toxic burden of chemicals, we are not feeding our bodies the proper nutrients, we are nutritional deficient, and some of us have little to no activity & these are some of the reasons why our bodies are becoming stagnant and increasingly polluted. It would be silly to take Motrin for a pebble stuck in your shoe when all you had to do was pluck it out. So why not on this journey go ahead, do some research and start addressing the issues at hand.

We are creating a perfect storm within our bodies. The less nutrients we consume, more toxins we add, create this world win of health issues. It's sad that our western diet is made up of red meats, vegetable oils, white flour and sugar. Who would have thought that something so simple as eating has become so complicated? Food does matter. It talks to your DNA. Food can change your DNA!

The foods you eat have a major impact your life — It affects your gut health and along with increasing or decreasing the inflammation in your body. Unfortunately, our western world diet are full of foods that have a bad impact on both your gut and your inflammation. If it was made in a lab, avoid it. Do a little research and you will find that our western diet that is made up of processed, fake foods, chemicals, sugar and corn oils are all highly flaming the fan of your inflammation.

We have a shortage of nutrients in our food system. The most common foods that you load up your grocery cart with are loaded with bad carbs, fillers, preservatives, additives, flavorings, and chemicals. Your body doesn't have any idea what do to with all this fake food. We are creating a weaker human race, inflammation and pain along with the possibility of welcoming other diseases and disorders. Your diet and lifestyle choices is what has caused any health issues that you may have unless you were born with a health issue then you can look at your parents diet , surroundings and lifestyle choices. It can go back generations. The only way to get back our health and vitality is to look at the root of it all.

You can change and control your life.

Think about what you're putting in your body. Either you're fighting disease or feeding disease. You must get a concept of nutrient density. Gluten, dairy and soy products create inflammation in the digestive tract. In ancient times grains were prepared by soaking, sprouting and fermenting but that tradition in making them been long forgotten with our fast-paced culture.

Let's talk more about store bought bread:

The bread you're buying at the store really isn't real bread you're buying. The white bread in the grocery is not the bread that our ancestors use to eat. 65% of the foods we eat are made from grains that are grown in a field such as grain bread, whiskey pasta and beer just to name a few. Wheat is made up of 3 parts the bran, the germ and the starchy endosperm.

The way the grain is processed has a huge impact not only on the way it taste and how healthy it is for you. Our ancestors used every part of the grain when they made their bread. White bread on the store shelves is made by an industrial process that strips out the wheat into all-purpose flour and in most cases if you read the back of the labels you will see chemicals additives added. These chemical additives is what gives white bread a longer shelve life.

White bread is also only made from the starchy endosperm which your body turns into pure sugar.

If you have inflammation in the digestive system undigested proteins leak into the blood stream creating a heightened immune reaction that often can lead to a leaky gut which causes other problems.

Most often than none, it's unrealistic for any lifestyle change to happen overnight. It does take practice but with practice does come change. Don't allow the bigger picture to discourage you. Every small thing you change to better your health will pay off in the end. It's the small steps that can make a big difference. Start by looking at your life and evaluating the toxins you may regularly come in contact with, understand what must take priority, and replace with these alternative options that I have listed in this article.

You have the power to make a difference in your life. You've always had the power. No one can force you to become more aware of what you put on your body and what you put in your body. What you eat is just as important as what you put on your body. Adjusting your life, reading labels and catering to your specific health needs isn't easy but it will benefit you in the long run. This is one of the smartest decisions that you can make. Not only will you start to look and feel better but think of the medical cost that you could be saving your future self.

Healthy Cells Grow From the Inside Out

Look into getting a Knowledgeable Health Practitioner:

The very first thing that you need to do is look into getting a knowledgeable holistic health practitioner!

The main reason why you should work with a knowledgeable health practitioner is its patient-centered medical healing at its best. Unfortunately, when it comes to your body there isn't a one size fits all approach to dealing with it and often times you are left still searching for the answers to your symptoms when all you want is your zest for life back. A knowledgeable health practitioner will care for you as an individual as they won't look at your body as a whole they will treat each individual body symptom, imbalance and dysfunction. They will take into consideration the whole person, including physical, mental and spiritual aspects, when treating a health condition or promoting wellness. I want you to understand that you are made up of interdependent parts and if one part is not working properly, all the other parts will be affected. A knowledgeable health practitioner certainly moves from the confusion of the "one size fits all treatment" approach that we know isn't working to the one that will cater to what your body needs. Let's not forget that each of us are a unique case and unless you get a proper thorough clinical evaluation, trying to figure what medical advise you need online is dubious at best.

In order to find your food code here are a list of things that need to be addressed in your life. When all these things are addressed and you are learning to know what your body needs and needs to avoid then you can find your personal food code. I never said it was going to be easy.

1. Address Food sensitivities

Food allergies

Many people are unaware that certain foods are actually working against their bodies. You should see a specialist and be tested to ensure you have no food allergies. Your lymphatic system can also be affected by your gut. If your gut is inflamed and not healed this is taxing on your immune system which in return is taxing on your lymphatic system. Consider adding prebiotics and probiotics to help support gut health along with eating properly and avoiding these common food allergens.

Common food allergens that can contribute to an inflamed gut are:

Nightshades

Eggs

Grains (gluten)

Dairy

Lugumes

If you allergic to certain foods it is will involve you're the immune system. You know that your immune system controls how your body defends itself. Your body see's inflammatory foods as invaders and will kick in your autoimmunity responses. For example if you have a food allergy to cow's milk, your immune system will see cow's milk as an invader. In-return your immune system overreacts by producing antibodies called Immunoglobulin E (IgE). These antibodies travel to cells that release chemicals, causing an allergic reaction to start fighting for your body. Being tested for food allergies seems to be easiest way to check to see if you have any food allergies so you can start avoiding these foods and help your immune system become strong again.

2. Address nutritional deficiencies

Having nutritional deficiencies certainly adds gas to the fire. When you are deficient it can aggravate the symptoms: vitamin D, iron, omega-3 fatty acids, selenium, zinc, copper, vitamin A, the B vitamins, and iodine.

3. Address Chronic Candida

Did you know that an overload of Candida was picked up at birth or shortly thereafter? We were supposed to be getting good friendly bacteria from our mother's at birth, but "our" mother's had Candida overgrowth and unknowing passed it on to us. And over the years, our bodies has become more and more compromised. Your gut microbes could be dramatically affecting your thyroid health. There is a lot of misinformation and misunderstanding about Candida. Both from the medical profession and on the internet. It is easy to get fooled into thinking, as many sites will try to convince you, that all anyone needs to do is to take their product or buy their e-book. Of course, they will all have testimonies. What they don't tell you in those testimonies is how the Candida came back — in a month or two or in six months. However long it took for the Candida to overgrow enough to start causing symptoms again. It is important to know that dealing with Candida is not an easy fix.

4. Address Hormonal imbalances

After researching many hours on this topic, I've found that where your body stores fat is hint to what is going on with you internally with your hormones. As our hormone levels change with age, pregnancy, exercise, eating habits, or other life events, fat adjusts itself to our every changing hormonal events and places itself in different area's in our body. Our hormones have a direct impact on how much body fat we store and where it is stored on our bodies. Wouldn't it be wonderful to know what approach to take to fix those thunder thighs or that muffin top? Now even with this information it's just a stepping stone of knowledge to better equip you a healthier you. This completely changes how you and what you should be eating.

Insomnia. It's amazing how the food we eat affects our health, sleep patterns and even our "gasp" sex drives. Unfortunately, when you don't get enough sleep, it can age us faster , cause depression, weight gain, make us forget things, gives us headaches and we have a greater chance of developing heart disease. If you have issues like snoring or sleep apnea and are overweight, one thing you can do is lower your body fat index. For those of us that don't have snoring or sleep apnea we ask the question," Sleep why you hate me so much!" We need to feed our bodies to get more, Tryptophan, serotonin and melatonin. (Serotonin is a brain chemical that helps you sleep) and melatonin (the hormone that makes you sleepy) Tryptophan is an essential amino acid, which means you have to get it from your diet because your body cannot produce it. Your body uses tryptophan to make the neurotransmitters serotonin and melatonin. Red Onion Tea helps with insomnia Directions

1 cup of water

1 onion, cut in quarters

Blend, strain and drink

Epsom salt bath which is rich in magnesium

Sleepy time Goats Milk Bath

2 cups of powdered goat's milk

2 cup of Epsom salt

1 cup of sea salt

2 cup of baking soda

10 drops of lavender essential oil

Combine the dry ingredients and the lavender essential oil. Store in a closed container. When you are ready to take a bath add 1 cup of dry ingredients. (Kids can use up to 1/2 cup of the mixture). Bathe 3 times weekly, soaking for at least 12 minutes.

Lavender has a reputation as a mild tranquilizer. Simply dab a bit of the oil onto your temples and forehead before you hit the pillow. The aroma should help send you off to sleep.

 Lastly, don't obsess over not sleeping. Studies have shown that people who worry about falling asleep have greater trouble falling asleep! It may help to remind yourself that while sleeplessness is a pain in the ass it isn't life-threatening. Let's try to be mellow-bellow. Eat foods that foods contribute to calmness and sleepiness.

5 plants to help you sleep better!

1. Aloe Vera — emits oxygen at night to help you combat insomnia and improve the overall sleep quality.

2. Lavender- Lavender is a plant that is well known to induce sleep and reduce anxiety. The smell of lavender slows down your heart rate and reduces anxiety levels.

3. Jasmine plant- The smell of jasmine has been shown to improve the quality of sleep.

4. English Ivy- it's beneficial for those who have breathing problems and asthma. Studies have shown that English ivy can reduce air molds to 94% in 12 hours.

5. Snake plant- emits oxygen into the night while you sleep, taking carbon dioxide from the air inside your home. It also filters nasty household toxins from the home.

Poor liver function due to the use of pharmaceuticals drugs.You really need to do research on your medications. Some medications have a negative effect on your lymph system and since estrogen is metabolized primarily in the liver try to not use pharmaceutical drugs unless absolutely necessary. If you must take these medications then try introducing liver-supporting supplements into your diet, such as cucumber juice, milk thistle extract, calcium d-glucarate, folic acid and taurine.https://www.lymphnet.org/membersOnly/dl/reprint/Vol_24/Vol_24-N4_Drugs_LE.pdf

Magnesium deficiencies Magnesium is necessary for metabolizing estrogen in the liver. Magnesium is a mineral that plays a important part in our health and well-being. It's one of the forgotten minerals and it's vital for many processes within the body. Magnesium helps to keep the nervous system healthy and to calm your nerves when you are stressed. In fact, did you know that magnesium is the first mineral depleted when you are stressed? So if you have any type of stress in your life magnesium is the first mineral that goes out the window. Magnesium is also an important mineral co-factor for enzymes that have biochemical reactions in the body. In other words it plays a large role in digestive system health as it helps enzymes do their job as well as to loosen the body to relax and ease to support the metabolic processes. These recipes are from my book AWARENESS HAS MAGIC.

Calming Magnesium Body Butter My homemade magnesium body butter will help replace the magnesium that our bodies need to thrive to survive. I always try to apply a little to my feet and shoulders before bed. This helps me relax and also get a fantastic night's sleep. It's pretty easy to make and the benefits are overwhelming. Magnesium deficiency is very common and it mimics other common symptoms and many other conditions like, being tired and felling run down, not sleeping well, getting headaches, gut issues, and even feeling stressed and anxious. Here is a list of things that can lower our magnesium levels:

Too much caffeine

Processed food and Sugar

Too much stress

Poor sleep habits

Calming Magnesium Body Butter

1/2 cup cocoa butter

1/2 cup of coconut oil and melt

1/4 cup magnesium oil

Add 10 drops of lavender essential oil,

Add 10 drops cedarwood essential oil

Add 10 drops frankincense essential oil

Place a heat-safe glass measuring cup/bowl inside a pot that has 1-2 inches of simmering water over medium heat. Add the cocoa butter and melt it in your double boiler until it's completely melted.

Remove the cocoa butter from heat, and add 1/2 cup extra virgin coconut oil to the melted cocoa butter and stir until completely the coconut oil has melted. Next add 1/4 cup magnesium oil to the mixture and combine. Place the mixture in the refrigerator to cool for about 30-60 minutes (until it is cooled completely). After the mixture has completely cooled and became a solid. Use a hand mixer or stand mixer to whip it. Start on low and increase speed slowly. Whip for about 3-5 minutes. Next add the 10 drops each of lavender essential oil, the 10 drops of cedar wood essential oil, and the 10 drops of frankincense essential oil. Scrape down the sides of the bowl and continue whipping for another 5 minutes or so, until the magnesium body butter is light and fluffy. The color of the magnesium body butter will change from yellow to a pale ivory and almost white color. Lastly put the magnesium body butter into mason jars and seal tightly with a lid. Make sure to label and date the top of the lid. This recipe makes enough for two 4 oz. glass jars.

Household chemicals. Did you know that it takes 26 seconds for the chemicals to enter into your bloodstream? The real reality is we are damaging our DNA and we are changing our genetic makeup for future generations. There was a study a few years back that said the umbilical cord of an average American baby has over 200 known chemicals in it. Eighty percent of the common chemicals that are used daily in this country, we know almost nothing about. Our children are being born toxic and we have no idea if these toxins are already doing some sort of damage their brains, their immune system, their reproductive system, and any other developing organs. Are we unknowingly setting ourselves up for failure in the womb, even before birth?

Scientists and researchers are concerned that many of these chemicals may be carcinogenic or wreak havoc with our hormones, our body's regulating system.

Most products have a warning label that is typed in bold "Keep out of Reach of Children". As consumers, we believe that if our children don't ingest these products they will not be harmed by them. This can be far from the truth. Think about other common methods of exposure are through the skin and our respiratory tract. WE are along with our children are often in contact with the chemical residues housecleaning products do leave behind, by crawling, lying and sitting on the freshly cleaned floor.

Scientists at Norway's University of Bergen tracked 6,000 people, with an average age of 34 at the time of enrollment in the study, who used the cleaning products over a period of two decades, according to the research published in the American Thoracic Society's American Journal of Respiratory and Critical Care Medicine.

These chemicals can chemicals bind together.

Exposure to phthalates has been associated with lower IQ levels.

These chemicals can also be found in the shampoos, conditioners, body sprays, hair sprays, perfumes, make up, cleaning supplies, colognes, soap and nail polish that we use.

The results follow a study by French scientists in September 2017 that found nurses who used disinfectants to clean surfaces at least once a week had a 24 percent to 32 percent increased risk of developing lung disease.

Scientists and researchers are concerned that many of these chemicals may be carcinogenic or wreak havoc with our hormones, our body's regulating system.

It's not enough to be aware of all the outdoor chemicals that we are exposed to everyday but inside our homes we can have more power and control. We have to be more aware about using chemical cleaners, paints, glues, body lotions, toothpastes, underarm deodorants, hair products and pesticides. Instead start to begin to use products that don't pollute our very own bodies. We must read labels, make our own products and do our own research. I can't stress this enough. We must take a stand for our health. Stop using commercial products that are laced with unknown and harmful body damaging products.

You can reduce your exposure to them by eating organic foods, making your own cleaning chemicals and using alternative pest control methods.

You can also find many great recipes for alternative cleaning solutions in my book AWARENESS HAS MAGIC.

Here are two recipes from my book **AWARENESS HAS MAGIC.**

Vanilla grapefruit linen spray

2-1/2 cups filtered water

3 drops pink grapefruit essential oil

2 drops vanilla essential oil

1/4 cup vodka

The vodka helps the water dry quickly after you spray it on your linens. Theses essential oils that are used create a beautifully fresh vanilla grapefruit scent that is perfect for a summer pick me up. This spray is very versatile. It can be used on clothing, fabric furniture, or even as a quick air freshener.

If the vodka smell is slightly strong just add another drop or two of essential oil.

Always shake the bottle be before spraying on your linen.

Tub & Tile Cleaner

1 /4 cup baking soda

1/4 cup lemon juice

Or 10 drops of lemon essential oil

3 Tablespoons Epsom salt

3 Tablespoons Sal Suds or Castile liquid soap

1/2 cup white vinegar

Pour the vinegar into the bottle, followed by the baking soda and Epsom salt. Shake the bottle to combine the ingredients. Add the Sal suds gently shaking the bottle to combine. Mix all ingredients in a bottle with a sealable lid.

Scrub and then rinse with water and wet clean rag.

5. Parasites and Heavy Metals

Heavy metals weaken our body's defense system against foreign invaders and make it convenient for them to set up house. American's are not being protected as we should from pollution. We don't have to go to a 3rd world country or even a foreign country be subjected to contaminated water which can led to illnesses.

The pollution in our air, water, food supply, cleaning products, body products, commercial weed killers and chem trails in our environment. It's really hard not to have some sort of health issues that come from a heavy metal over load on our bodies. Just imagine commercial meat production, can goods and prepackaged foods. Heavy metals make a very acid environment which is very harmful to your gut flora where parasites and candida love to flourish. Candida and parasites actually do serve a purpose in your body they are to protect us from the potentially fatal complications of heavy metal poisoning. They feed on heavy metals and store them within biofilms- buffering us from heavy metal overload.

Do you find that you are developing new allergies as you become older; are you always tired, do you have poor digestion, gas, heartburn; sugar cravings, are you irritable, frequent headaches; poor memory, "fogged in" feeling, dizziness, recurring depression, vaginal infections, menstrual difficulties, urinary tract infections, infertility, hay fever, postnasal drip, habitual coughing, catch colds easily, sore throat, athlete's foot, skin rash, psoriasis, cold extremities, arthritis-like symptoms, do you feel miserable in general? If answered yes to most of these symptoms then should be tested for candidiasis.

According to the publication in 1995 "Parasitic Diseases" it states the following rate of infection per species.

Nematodes (Round Worms)	1 billion individuals
Cestodes (Tape Worms)	300 million individuals
Tremadodes (Flukes)	300 million individuals
Protozoa (Amoebas)	1 billion individuals
Arthropods (Insects parasites)	500 million individuals

How can I start to detox from Parasites and Heavy Metals?

Each per-son is different and I encour-age you to seek out a qual-i-fied nutri-tion-ist or other qualified healthcare practitioner in order to assess exactly which nutri-ents, herbs, homeopathic and nat-ural reme-dies and/or in which com-bi-na-tion that will help you achieve your goal. No one treatment is the same since we all have different diary needs, illness's and lift styles. Getting the root cause of your issues are the main objective. I strongly recommend you get with your health care provider and allow them to schedule you for further tested if needed. This is how   and where you will figure your own personal food code.

6. Heal your Gut

Your gut is your portal to health. It houses 80 percent of your immune system, and without your gut being healthy it is practically impossible to have a healthy immune system. A leaky gut have been linked to hormonal imbalances, autoimmune diseases such as rheumatoid arthritis and Hashimotos thyroiditis, diabetes, chronic fatigue, fibromyalgia, anxiety, depression, eczema and rosacea, and that is just to name a few. So you can understand why a properly working digestive system (your gut) is vital to your health. Contrary to what we use to believe. We now know that having a leaky gut is one of the main reasons, and probably the beginning stage, for developing an autoimmune disease. Having a leaky gut means that the tight junctions that usually hold the walls of your intestines together have become loose, allowing undigested food particles, microbes, toxins, and more to leave your gut and enter your bloodstream. This will cause your body to become full of inflammation, which in return will start to trigger an autoimmune condition and if you already have an autoimmune condition it will certainly make it worse. Luckily for you. Your gut is made up of wonderful cells that can turn over very quickly, so you can start to heal your gut in as little as thirty days, by following these 4 R guidelines: Remove, Restore, Replace and Repair

Remove the damage — Remove these inflammatory foods, household & body chemicals, drink filtered water(to avoid fluoride and chloride) , stop using aluminum brand deodorant, start using fluoride free brand tooth pastes, start to reduce your stress that damage your gut, do a detox to heal any gut infections from yeast, parasites, or bacteria.

Restore the Strong — replenish the enzymes and digestive acids that are necessary for proper digestion

Replace with friendly Bacteria — Make sure you are taking plenty a good strong probiotic that is full of these much needed "good bacteria" to start supporting your immune system. Here is a great product that I use. You can do your own research and I am sure there are other brands out there that are wonderful too. Garden Of Life Dr. Formulated Probiotics Once Daily Women's, 30 Count

Repair the digestive Tract — Give you gut a fighting chance by supplying the nutrients and amino acids needed to build a healthy gut lining. (Gelatin can improve your ability to produce adequate gastric acid secretions that are needed for proper digestion and nutrient absorption. Glycine from gelatin is important for restoring a healthy mucosal lining in the stomach and facilitating with the balance of digestive enzymes (Here is a brand that I use   Garden of Life RAW Enzymes Women, 90 Capsules) and stomach acid. The best way to consume gelatin make them into broth or soup. You can do this by simply brewing some bone broth at home using this Bone Broth Recipe.

Throughout my latest book, you will find useful, informative and easy to understand recipes for your mind, body and spirit. When I started writing this book, I wanted to introduce you to the idea of a cleaner less toxic world and for you to learn just how simply easy it is for you to start creating your own cleaning recipes throughout your home but this book has transformed into so much more than just a book full of all natural DIY recipes.

This book will enlighten you and help you have a deeper understanding of not only why you should be more aware but how to be more aware. AWARENESS HAS MAGIC.

There is no one size fits all with Hypothyroidism

I started to research to begin to try to understand that there's really not a one size fits all for us with hypothyroidism but there are certain ways we can eat, things that we need to start incorporating and things we need to start avoiding that will certainly help begin the healing process. Diet alone wasn't enough to help my body start fighting this battle that is raging in your body. I needed to start addressing other areas in your life that can cause inflammation like Dietary Allergies, Addressing gut health and avoiding Chemical toxins and endocrine disruptors. In this book, I have gone in to detail many times over to explain and help guide you on your journey. I am sharing things that I've learned along the way to help you have a smoother transaction that I did. I hope you are taking notes, highlighting and writing along the side of the book. Not everything in this book will affect you directly but it might others. Food is very important part of the healing process. Food not just calories it is information. It talks to your DNA and tells it what to do. My most powerful tool to change my health was my fork. I needed to stop going long periods of time without food. My body always needed energy. If my blood sugar starts to drop this creates a stress reaction and now your adrenal glands will do what it needs to do to maintain my body's function by releasing more cortisol or adrenaline. Eating often would help put your body back in its normal cycle. You need to eat foods that nourish your body and not hinder it.

I really had no idea how powerful food really was until after I was diagnosed with Hypothyroidism. Many people with hypothyroidism are deficient in Magnesium, B-12, Zinc, Iodine, B2, Vitamin C, Selenium, Vitamin D and Vitamin A.

The Standard American diet in a nutshell is loaded with unhealthy saturated and Tran's fats. Our meals are unbalanced, over-sized and loaded with sugar, salt, artificial ingredients and preservatives. We have an abundance of food at our finger tips but yet we are extremely malnourished and mineral deficient. We are literally starving our bodies to death! People are not obtaining the basic nutrients their bodies needs in order to fuel what is needed to perform its proper functions. We are literally running on empty! There is about 20 million estimated Americans with some type of hypothyroid disorder.

Although my thyroid is small, it produces a hormone that influences every cell, tissue and organ in the body. My thyroid determines the rate in which my body produces the energy from nutrients and oxygen. So I need to start eating foods that fed my thyroid. I needed to start nourishing my body back to health with foods that jump kicked my metabolism too. After being diagnosed my priorities were made clearer. I had to start listening to my body, stop taking my health for granted and continuing to research to figure out what I needed to do to "fix me". I started making my own cleaning products, lotions and deodorant's. Our skin is the largest organ in our body and it absorbs everything we put on it.

Final Thoughts:

Hypothyroidism is the kind of disease that carries a bit of mystery with it. This book is not for readers looking for quick answers. There is not one size fits all. You have to be in charge of your health. I didn't write my books to sell you any "snake oil" in a bottle. I've written my books to be an eye opener for you and to share with you what I have learned on my journey. The solutions in this new book will help many people if you start applying the methods and listen with an open ear. There are many incredible holistic practitioners, authors and researchers with experience and expertise in this area. I've done my best to pull from all their expertise, as well as my own knowledge and clinical experience. I want to make it easy for you to find the answers quickly, all in the one place, because I'm all too familiar with that awful side effects of hypothyroidism. I certainly don't want you to have to spend years finding solutions, like I did. I also what you to understand that there isn't an easy "one pill" solution, but the "one pill" approach that our current medical system is using is NOT WORKING because the underlying cause for hypothyroidism is not being addressed.

I am SO GRATEFUL and MOVED by all of you who are reaching out to me on this JOURNEY and I want to give back to you all. My way of doing so is to allow you to see a glimpse of my true essence and share with you what I hope will be inspiring for at least some of you.

People act as though 46 is old. I say it's as young or as old as you allow yourself to be. And just as a fine wine, we can get better with age. I know, for me, I feel the best now in body, mind and spirit than ever before and I want to share with you why.

For most of my life, I was clueless as to my purpose (other than being a Mom, friend and a wife). I have been in multiple relationships w/ the wrong men, wrong friendships, stayed at a job I dreaded going to each day and was basically just going through the motions in my life without passion or excitement. I was giving in to my fear with each of these choices and I was living a life of not being true to my inner being.

We all have some parts of us that have held us back from not having the ultimate life, body, health, relationships, finances that I wanted. I have learned in my journey that it is up to us to figure out what part of us is in resistance to it. What part of us is giving in to FEAR of something?

I am FINALLY at a place in my life where I recognize the reoccurring choices I've made in my life based on fear that have prevented me from having the life I want

– and am committed to listening to my intuition and my heart and creating the life of my dreams.

At 45, I am now living consciously and honoring my true inner being. Even though fear still rises its head, I choose not to allow it to dictate any more of my life.

I am finally living my purpose with passion of helping others to change the beliefs/mindsets/habits that are holding them back from having the body/weight/energy/health and life that they want.

So, my friends, no matter your age, don't let fear guide your decisions and open yourselves up to the life that you were destined to have. Only through acknowledging the fear and choosing faith instead is the secret to living your greatest life possible.

MESSAGE FROM THE AUTHOR: A.L. Childers

MESSAGE FROM THE AUTHOR

Sometimes in life we just need clarity. You have to step out of your comfort zone and focus on where your path is headed. You were born with the capacity of abundance. You need to clear away any of the emotional, mental and energetic debris that is in the way of your ability to see who you really are in order to create the life you really deserve. My goal in this book is to help you understand and show you how easy it is for you to start cutting out the foods that don't nourish your body. Hypothyroidism is a very tricky condition and complicated disorder to manage. The foods we eat can interfere with your treatment. Our body is lacking certain nutrients that heavily influence the function of our thyroid gland while certain foods can inhibit your body's ability to absorb the replacement hormones. There is no one size fits all program when you are dealing with hypothyroidism. When you start to eat smarter and are aware of what foods feed your body, despite the condition, you can start to feel better and manage your symptoms. Americans are in such a pathetic health crisis. We have the abundance of everything at our finger tips but yet we 1 in 3 people are on some sort of medication. It doesn't matter if it's Prescribed or over the counter. Why are we are in such a state of denial? Every Cell in your body responds to the foods you eat, the products you put on your body to the house hold chemicals that you purchase for your home. All of these things have a direct impact on your hormones and in return your hormones have a direct impact on every major system in your body. Not to mention that our body is lacking certain nutrients that heavily influence the function of every cell in our body. The foods that we consume, oh, the foods we consume. It is my immense pleasure to write another book on hypothyroidism. In this age of overly processed, genetically modified, artificially flavored and preservative loaded foods. It's no wonder that more people are wanting to eat a more wholesome and a more all natural diet. We are trying to find our way back to the basics. I hope this book encourages you and inspires you to seek out the truth and start healing your body from the inside out. All I can give you is the blueprint of things you can start doing today to incorporate a healthier you. I am living this way. I can talk about what has worked for me and share my knowledge with you. Taking charge of your health doesn't have to be complicated. The journey has just begun. Each day is filled with the opportunity to make an impact and have that ripple effect with your health. My mission is to do everything in my power to start to heal and reach your fullest potential. To help be a source of inspiration you seek and attract what you desire with the faith that your vision of success is your destiny! You deserve to be healthy. You have the power and you have the mindset. Never forget: What we eat, governs what we become. Success is getting what you want. Happiness is wanted what you get.

professional. I am not a doctor, or a medical professional. This book is designed for as an educational and entertainment tool only. Please always check with your health practitioner before taking any vitamins, supplements, or herbs, as they may have side-effects, especially when combined with medications, alcohol, or other vitamins or supplements. Knowledge is power, educate yourself and find the answer to your health care needs. Wisdom is a wonderful thing to seek. I hope this book will teach and encourage you to take leaps in your life to educate yourself for a happier & healthier life. You have to take ownership of your health

References:

Thakre D, Rayalu S, Kawade R, Meshram S, Subrt J, Labhsetwar N. Magnesium incorporated bentonite clay for defluoridation of drinking water. Journal of Hazardous Materials. 2010 August 15;180(1-3):122-30. doi: 10.1016/j.jhazmat.2010.04.001.

Cusumano V, Rossano F, Merendino RA, Arena A, Costa GB, ancuso G, Baroni A, Losi E. Immunobiological activities of mould products: functional impairment of human monocytes exposed to aflatoxin B1. Research in Microbiology. 1996 June:147(5):385-91.

Julia R. Barrett. Liver Cancer and Aflatoxin: New Information from the Kenyan Outbreak. Environmental Health Perspectives. December 2005; 113(12): A837-A838.

Thieu NQ, Ogie B, Pettersson H. Efficacy of bentonite clay in ameliorating aflatoxicosis in piglets fed aflatoxin contaminated diets. Tropical Animal Health and Production. 2008 December;40(8):649-56. doi: 10.1007/s11250-008-9144-3.

Zaitan H, Bianchi D, Achak O, Charik T. A comparative study of the adsorption and desorption of o-xylene onto bentonite clay and alumina. Journal of Hazardous Materials. 2008 May 1;153(1-2):852-9.

Günister E, Isci S, Oztekin N, Erim FB, Ece OI, Gungor N. Effect of cationic surfactant adsorption on the rheological and surface properties of bentonite dispersions. Journal of Colloid and Interface Science. 2006 November 1;303(1):137-41.

Jarup L. Hazards of heavy metal contamination. British Medical Bulletin. 2003;68:167-82.

Oyanedel-Craver VA, Fuller M, Smith JA. Simultaneous sorption of benzene and heavy metals onto two organoclays. Journal of Colloid and Interface Science. 2007 May 15;309(2):485-92.

Martyn T. Smith. Advances in Understanding Benzene Health Effects and Susceptibility. Annual Review of Public Health. Vol. 31: 133-148. April 2010. DOI: 10.1146/annurev.publhealth.012809.103646.

Gitipour S, Bowers MT, Bodocsi A. The Use of Modified Bentonite for Removal of Aromatic Organics from Contaminated Soil. Journal of Colloid and Interface Science. 1997 December 15;196(2):191-198.

Ibrahim IK, Shareef AM, Al-Joubory KM. Ameliorative effects of sodium bentonite on phagocytosis and Newcastle disease antibody formation in broiler chickens during aflatoxicosis. Research in Veterinary Science. 2000 October;69(2):119-22.

https://www.fda.gov/Drugs/DrugSafety/ucm483838.htm

https://www.bulkherbstore.com/Bentonite-Clay-Powder/

https://en.wikipedia.org/wiki/Bentonite

^ Jump up to: a b Odom, I. E. (1984). "Smectite clay Minerals: Properties and Uses". Philosophical Transactions of the Royal Society A: Mathematical, Physical and Engineering Sciences. 311 (1517): 391. Bibcode:1984RSPTA.311..391O. doi:10.1098/rsta.1984.0036. JSTOR 37332.

Jump up ^ Theng, B.K.G. 1979. Formation and Properties of Clay Polymer Complexes. Developments in Soil Science 9. Elsevier, Amsterdam, ISBN 0-444-41706-0

Jump up ^ Lagaly G., 1995. Surface and interlayer reactions: bentonites as adsorbents. pp. 137–144, in Churchman, G.J., Fitzpatrick, R.W., Eggleton R.A. Clays Controlling the Environment. Proceedings of the 10th International Clay Conference, Adelaide, Australia. CSIRO Publishing, Melbourne, ISBN 0-643-05536-3

Jump up ^ R.H.S, Robertson, 1986. Fuller's Earth. A History of calcium montmorillonite. Volturna, Press, U.K., ISBN 0-85606-070-4

Jump up ^ Guyonnet, Dominique; Gaucher, Eric; Gaboriau, Hervé; Pons, Charles-Henri; Clinard, Christian; Norotte, VéRonique; Didier, GéRard (2005). "Geosynthetic Clay Liner Interaction with

Leachate: Correlation between Permeability, Microstructure, and Surface Chemistry". Journal of Geotechnical and Geoenvironmental Engineering. 131 (6): 740. doi:10.1061/(ASCE)1090-0241(2005)131:6(740).

Jump up ^ Potassium bentonite. McGraw-Hill Dictionary of Scientific and Technical Terms. Retrieved June 12, 2008. Answers.com

Jump up ^ Karnland, O., Olsson, S. and Nilsson, U. 2006. Mineralogy and sealing properties of various bentonites and smectite-rich clay materials. SKB Technical Report TR-06-30. Stockholm, Sweden. [1]

Jump up ^ Bentonite Archived August 1, 2009, at the Wayback Machine. from oregonstate.edu website

Jump up ^ [2] from Official Journal of the European Resuscitation Council

Jump up ^ "FDA warns consumers about health risks with Alikay Naturals – Bentonite Me Baby – Bentonite Clay". Drugs: Drug Safety and Availability. USFDA. 29 January 2016. Retrieved 30 January 2016.

Jump up ^ DrugBank

Jump up ^ "Database of Select Committee on GRAS Substances (SCOGS) Reviews Bentonite". FDA database. FDA. Retrieved 15 August 2011.

Jump up ^ Noble, A. D., Ruaysoongnern, S., Penning de Vries, F. W. T., Hartmann, C. and Webb, M. J. 2004. Enhancing the agronomic productivity of degraded soils in North-east Thailand through clay-based interventions. In Seng, V., E. Craswell, S. Fukai, and K. Fischer, eds., Water and Agriculture, Proceedings No. 116, ACIAR, Canberra, pp. 147–160.

Jump up ^ Suzuki, Shinji; Noble, Andrew; Ruaysoongnern, Sawaeng; Chinabut, Narong (2007). "Improvement in Water-Holding Capacity and Structural Stability of a Sandy Soil in Northeast Thailand". Arid Land Research and Management. 21: 37. doi:10.1080/15324980601087430.

Jump up ^ Saleth, R.M., Inocencio, A., Noble, A.D., and Ruaysoongnern, S. 2009. Improving Soil Fertility and Water Holding Capacity with Clay Application: The Impact of Soil Remediation Research in Northeast Thailand. IWMI Research Report (in Review).

Jump up ^ Noble, A. D.; Gillman, G. P.; Nath, S.; Srivastava, R. J. (2001). "Changes in the surface charge characteristics of degraded soils in the wet tropics through the addition of beneficiated bentonite". Australian Journal of Soil Research. 39 (5): 991. doi:10.1071/SR00063.

Jump up ^ "Diaphragm wall". Retrieved 18 May 2014.

^ Jump up to: a b Gutberle (1994). "Slurry Walls". Virginia Tech. Archived from the original on 2012-01-05. Retrieved 2012-01-05. CS1 maint: BOT: original-url status unknown (link)

Jump up ^ T. Brown et al. 2013. World Mineral Production 2007-11. British Geological Survey, Nottingham, England. http://www.bgs.ac.uk/mineralsuk/statistics/worldArchive.html

1) Cooper DS. Subclinical Hypothyroidism. NEJM. 2001 Jul 26;345: 260– 265.

(2) Persky VW, Turyk ME, Wang L, Freels S, Chatterton R Jr, Barnes S, Erdman J Jr, Sepkovic DW, Bradlow HL, Potter S. Effect of soy protein on endogenous hormones in postmenopausal women. Am J Clin Nutr. 2002 Jan; 75(1): 145– 153. Erratum in: Am J Clin Nutr. 2002 Sep; 76(3): 695

(3) Toscano V, Conti FG, Anastasi E, Mariani P, Tiberti C, Poggi M, Montuori M, Monti S, Laureti S, Cipolletta E, Gemme G, Caiola S, Di Mario U, Bonamico M. Importance of gluten in the induction of endocrine autoantibodies and organ dysfunction in adolescent celiac patients. Am J Gastroenterol. 2000 Jul; 95(7): 1742–1748.

(4) Ellingsen DG, Efskind J. Effects of low mercury vapour exposure on the thyroid function in chloralkali workers. J Appl Toxicol. 2000 Nov– Dec; 20(6): 483– 489.

(5) Galletti PM, Joyet G. Effect of fluorine on thyroidal iodine metabolism in hyperthyroidism. J Clin Endocrinol Metab. 1958 Oct; 18(10): 1102– 1110.

(6) WJ, Pan Y; Johnson AR, et al. Reduction of chemical sensitivity by means of heat depuration, physical therapy and nutritional supplementation in a controlled environment. J Nutr Env Med. 1996;6: 141– 148.

(7) Pelletier C, Imbeault P, Tremblay A. Energy balance and pollution by organochlorines and polychlorinated biphenyls. Obes Rev. 2003 Feb; 4(1): 17– 24. Review.

(8) Bland J. Nutritional Endocrinology, Normalizing Hypothalamus-Pituitary-Thyroid Axis Function, 2002 Seminar Series Syllabus.

(9) Gaby AR. Sub-laboratory hypothyroidism and the empirical use of Armour thyroid. Altern Med Rev. 2004 Jun; 9(2): 157– 179.

(10) Goglia F. Biological effects of 3,5-diiodothyronine (T(2)). Biochemistry (Moscow). 2005 Feb; 70(2): 164– 172.

https://www.ncbi.nlm.nih.gov/pmc/articles/PMC2819418/

https://www.ncbi.nlm.nih.gov/pmc/articles/PMC2515351/

https://www.mindbodygreen.com/0-24663/9-lifestyle-changes-i-always-recommend-to-patients-with-autoimmune-diseases.html

https://draxe.com/digestive-enzymes/

https://draxe.com/recipe/beef-bone-broth/

https://www.ncbi.nlm.nih.gov/pubmed/22109896

http://www.ewg.org/tap-water/

http://www.who.int/mediacentre/factsheets/fs313/en/

http://www.who.int/ceh/capacity/Pesticides.pdf

https://www.ncbi.nlm.nih.gov/pmc/articles/PMC2665673/

http://www.endocrineweb.com/conditions/hypothyroidism/symptoms-hypothyroidism

http://www.healthnutnation.com/2013/11/07/10-ways-naturally-stimulate-digestive-fire/

http://www.balancingbrainchemistry.co.uk/peter-smith/26/GABA-Deficient-Anxiety.html

http://www.chrisbeatcancer.com/rebounding/

http://thyroid.about.com/od/symptomsrisks/a/All-About-Goitrogens-thyroid.htm

http://healthyeating.sfgate.com/oat-bran-vs-rolled-oats-1761.html

http://healthyeating.sfgate.com/benefits-raw-pumpkin-seeds-6627.html

http://healthylivinghowto.com/1/post/2013/02/what-to-do-about-high-cortisol.html

http://www.mayoclinic.org/healthy-lifestyle/nutrition-and-healthy-eating/in-depth/water/art-20044256

https://bragg.com/products/bragg-organic-apple-cider-vinegar.html

GENLAB Medical Diagnostics and Research Laboratory,

1 Marmara University, Engineering Faculty, Department of Chemical Engineering,

2 Marmara University, School of Physical Education and Sports – Istanbul,

3 University of Gaziantep, The School of Physical Education and Sports,

4 Firat University Medicine Faculty Biochemistry Department,

5 Muğla University The School of Physical Education and Sports, Mugla – Turkey

Correspondence to: Yrd. Doc. Dr. Kursat Karacabey, PhD

University of Gaziantep, The School of Physical Education

and Sports (Beden Egitimi ve Spor Y.O)

TR 27100, Gaziantep, TURKEY

FAX: +90 342 3600751

TEL:+90 342 3601616 Ext:1412 / 1417

EMAIL: kkaracabey@gmail.com

karacabey@gantep.edu.tr

Thyroid hormones and the interrelationship of cortisol and prolactin; Influence of prolonged, exhaustive exercise

http://www.ncbi.nlm.nih.gov/pubmed/19753538

Hypothyroid myopathy. Physiopathological approach.

http://www.ncbi.nlm.nih.gov/pubmed/1339062

Thyroid hormonal responses to intensive interval versus steady state endurance exercise sessions.

http://www.ncbi.nlm.nih.gov/pubmed/?term=thyroid+hormonal+responses+to+intensive+interval+exercise

Decreased serum T3 after an exercise session is independent of glucocorticoid peak

http://www.ncbi.nlm.nih.gov/pubmed/23918684

A review of effects of hypothyroidism on vascular transport in skeletal muscle during exercise

http://www.ncbi.nlm.nih.gov/pubmed/9018403

Human mitochondrial transcription factor (A) reduction and mitochondrial dysfunction in

hashimoto's hypothyroid myopathy

http://www.ncbi.nlm.nih.gov/pubmed/?term=human+mitochondrial+transcription+a+reduction+and+mitochondrial+dysfunction++in+Hashimoto%27s

http://www.thyroid.org/iodine-deficiency/

https://ods.od.nih.gov/factsheets/Iodine-HealthProfessional/

https://www.healthfulelements.com/blog/2015/09/your-thyroid-copper

https://www.westonaprice.org/health-topics/modern-diseases/copper-zinc-imbalance-unrecognized-consequence-of-plant-based-diets-and-a-contributor-to-chronic-fatigue/

http://www.webmd.com/diet/iron-rich-foods

Zimmermann MB, Köhrle J. The impact of iron and selenium deficiencies on iodine and thyroid metabolism: biochemistry and relevance to public health. Thyroid. 2002 Oct;12(10):867-78.

2. Triggiani V, Tafaro E, Giagulli VA, et al. Role of iodine, selenium and other micronutrients in thyroid function and disorders. Endocr Metab Immune Disord Drug Targets. 2009 Sep;9(3):277-94. Epub 2009 Sep 1.

3.   Zimmermann MB. The influence of iron status on iodine utilization and thyroid function. Annu Rev Nutr. 2006;26:367-89.

4.   Casgrain A, Collings R, Harvey LJ, et al. Effect of iron intake on iron status: a systematic review and meta-analysis of randomized controlled trials. Am J Clin Nutr. 2012 Oct;96(4):768-80. Epub 2012 Aug 29.

http://www.webmd.com/diet/iron-rich-foods#2

https://www.ncbi.nlm.nih.gov/pmc/articles/PMC2819418/

https://www.ncbi.nlm.nih.gov/pmc/articles/PMC2515351/

https://www.mindbodygreen.com/0-24663/9-lifestyle-changes-i-always-recommend-to-patients-with-autoimmune-diseases.html

https://draxe.com/digestive-enzymes/

https://draxe.com/recipe/beef-bone-broth/

https://www.ncbi.nlm.nih.gov/pubmed/22109896

http://www.ewg.org/tap-water/

http://www.who.int/mediacentre/factsheets/fs313/en/

http://www.who.int/ceh/capacity/Pesticides.pdf

https://www.ncbi.nlm.nih.gov/pmc/articles/PMC2665673/

http://whfoods.org/genpage.php?tname=dailytip&dbid=337

http://sleepfoundation.org/how-sleep-works/how-much-sleep-do-we-really-need

↑ http://www.mayoclinic.org/healthy-lifestyle/adult-health/expert-answers/sleep-and-weight-gain/faq-20058198

http://www.rd.com/slideshows/foods-that-help-you-sleep/#slideshow=slide7

http://www.webmd.com/sleep-disorders/excessive-sleepiness-10/10-results-sleep-loss?page=2

Source: Journal of the American College of Cardiology, 2004; PLOS ONE, 2009; Sleep Medicine Reviews, 2012

Source: Journal of Clinical Endocrinology & Metabolism, 2012; PLOS Medicine, 2004; Nature Communications, 2013; PNAS, 2013

Source: Headache, 2003; Headache, 2005

Howatson G, Bell PG, Tallent J, Middleton B, McHugh MP, Ellis J. Effect of tart cherry juice (Prunus cerasus) on melatonin levels and enhanced sleep quality. Eur J Nutr. 2011 Oct 30 [Epub ahead of print].

2. Pigeon WR, Carr M, Gorman C, Perlis ML. Effects of tart cherry juice beverage on the sleep of older adults with insomnia: a pilot study. Journal of Medicinal Food. 2010;13:579-583.

3. Centers for Disease Control and Prevention. "Unhealthy sleep-related behaviors – 12 states, 2009." Morbidity and Mortality Weekly Report. March 4, 2011 / 60(08);233-238. http://www.cdc.gov/mmwr/preview/mmwrhtml/mm6008a2.htm

4. Hossain JL, Shapiro CM. The prevalence, cost implications, and management of sleep disorders: an overview. Sleep and Breathing. 2002;6:85-102.

http://nutritiondata.self.com/foods-000079000000000000000.html

Dietary Guidelines for Americans – 2005. Washington, DC. US Dept of Health and Human Services and US Dept of Agriculture: 2005.

Ooka H, Segall PE, Timiras PS (January 1978). "Neural and endocrine development after chronic tryptophan deficiency in rats: II. Pituitary-thyroid axis". Mech. Ageing Dev. 7 (1): 19–24.

Koopmans SJ, Ruis M, Dekker R, Korte M (October 2009). "Surplus dietary tryptophan inhibits stress hormone kinetics and induces insulin resistance in pigs". Physiology & Behavior 98 (4): 402–410.

2011 NLN Position Paper on Exercises

2011 NLN Position Paper on Screening and Measurement for Early Detection of Breast Cancer Related Lymphedema

2011 NLN Position Paper on the Diagnosis and Treatment of Lymphedema

2013 ISL Consensus Document for the Diagnosis and Treatment of Lymphedema

Information about Lymphedema

Lymphedema Framework: International Consensus for the best practice for the management of lymphedema

Lymphedema: Overview

Treatments for Lymphedema

Detox, General Health, Healing, Health Concerns, Natural Remedies, Nutrition, SupplementationSigns of A Clogged Lymphatic System and 10 Ways To Cleanse ItMarch 8, 2016 | Derek Henry39.5k8346221546

https://www.ncbi.nlm.nih.gov/pubmed/10656352

https://growyouthful.com/remedy/enzymes-digestive.php

https://wordpress.com/post/thehypothyroidismchick.com/19708

https://www.lymphnet.org/membersOnly/dl/reprint/Vol_24/Vol_24-N4_Drugs_LE.pdf

https://www.sakara.com/blogs/mag/115709701-everything-you-need-to-know-about-your-lymphatic-system

Dee Anna Glaser, MD, professor of dermatology, St. Louis University; president, International Hyperhidrosis Society.Patricia Farris, MD, clinical assistant professor of dermatology, Tulane University; member, American Academy of Dermatology.

Eric Schweiger, MD, dermatologist; clinical instructor of dermatology, Mt. Sinai School of Medicine, New York Cit